4 Four Weeks to Fabulous

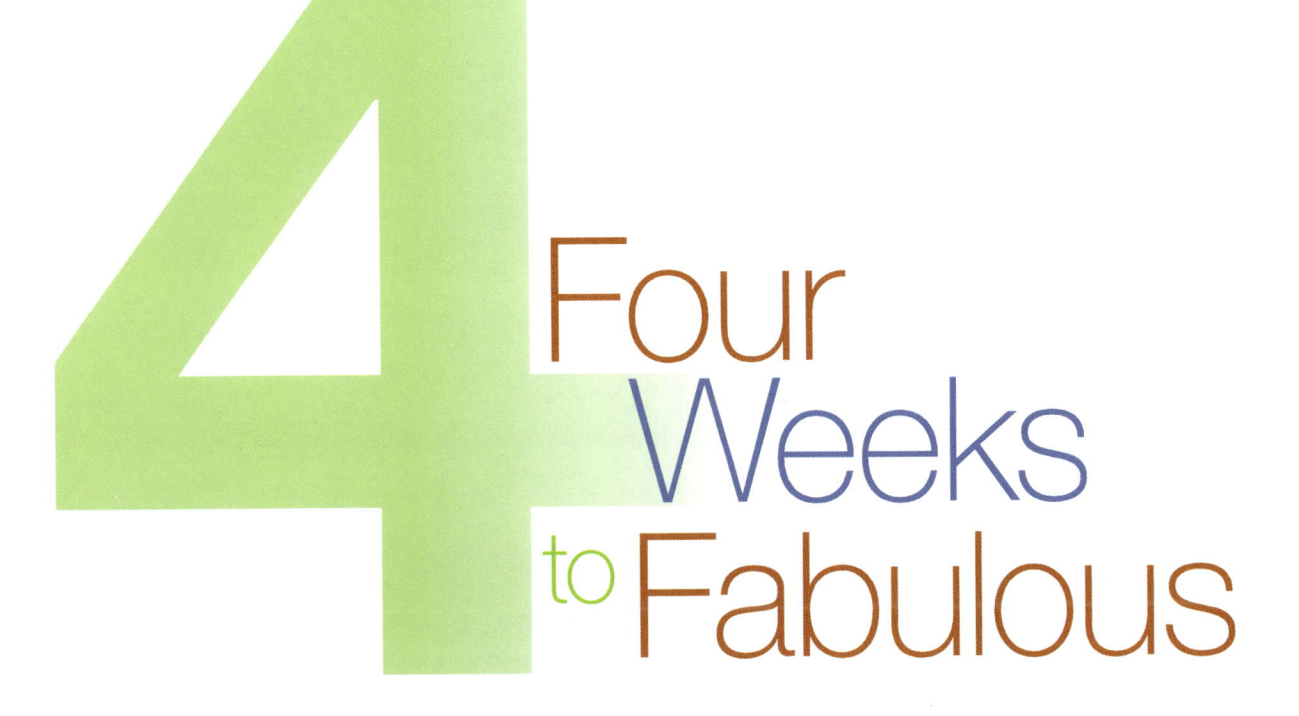

ALICE BURRON

Copyright © 2010 Alice Burron
All rights reserved.

ISBN: 1452867348
ISBN-13: 9781452867342
Library of Congress Control Number: 2010907642

This publication contains the opinions and ideas of its author. Every effort has been made to ensure the accuracy and clarity of the information contained; however, neither the author nor the publisher assumes any responsibility for errors, omissions, or changes that occur after publication. This book is sold with the understanding that the author is not rendering professional advice or service to the individual reader. The ideas and suggestions in this book are not intended as a substitute for consulting with your physician. The author specifically disclaims all responsibility for any liability, loss, or risk, personal or otherwise, which is incurred as a consequence, directly or indirectly, of the use and application of any of the contents of this book. Every effort has been made by the author to include recipes that have not been previously copyrighted. Should any such recipe appear in this book, it is without the author's knowledge and is unintentional.

Keeping your weight under control is not an accident—it's a gift that only you can give yourself.

Quiz: Are *You* Ready for Fabulous?

1. **You picked up this book because:**
    a) I want to get in shape so that I can look good and feel my best.
    b) I can't seem to gather the motivation to get moving, and hope that maybe this book will be the ticket to looking and feeling better.
    c) It was a total impulse purchase. The cover was so colorful and inspiring I just couldn't resist!

2. **How much of yourself are you willing to put into the Four Weeks To Fabulous routine?**
    a) 90-100% I'm so ready to feel fabulous!
    b) 80-90% I'm ready, but expect some obstacles.
    c) 50-70% My mind says I need to get up but my body wants to finish *CSI Miami* first.

3. **What kind of activities do you like to do most?**
    a) Structured, strength-building activities that may be hard but will give me awesome results.
    b) Activities that may be challenging but won't leave me sore in the morning.
    c) Something super-easy that will hopefully give me good results in a short amount of time.

4. **How do you prefer to exercise?**
    a) With friends or in a group so I have built in cheerleaders!
    b) With maybe one friend or a spouse, since we want to get in shape together.
    c) Alone. That way no one can tell if I mess up—or maybe skip a couple sit-ups.

5. **Are you willing to give up some of your favorite high-fat snacks for things that are a little more nutritious?**
    a) Sure. Make over my diet!
    b) It may be hard to give up some of the things I love to eat.
    c) I'm not really that thrilled about giving up my admittedly unhealthy snacks and drinks… are there any tasty *and* healthy foods out there?

The Results Are In!

1. Mostly A's: You're totally ready to get started on the Four Weeks to Fabulous Program! It's time to throw out your Twinkies and stock up on fruits and veggies. Get ready to see some results!

2. Mostly B's: You're fairly ready to get started. It might be helpful to do the program with a friend or spouse for encouragement and motivation. Plus, this way, they'll keep you accountable. If you stick with the program you'll see fabulous results in just four weeks!

3. Mostly C's: You haven't bought into this whole "exercise" thing yet, but you bought this book anyway. Maybe it was fate, or you knew you needed to get on track. Good for you! It might be difficult to throw out the unhealthy things in your lifestyle, but it will definitely be worth it in the end (and the rear end as well!).

Consider this: If you follow this program you will likely lose at least six pounds of body fat and noticeably increase your cardiovascular endurance and strength—enough to run a 5K without injury! Not bad considering all you are doing is giving your body the attention it deserves for four weeks!

Four Weeks to Fabulous
A Four-Week Journey to Better Health

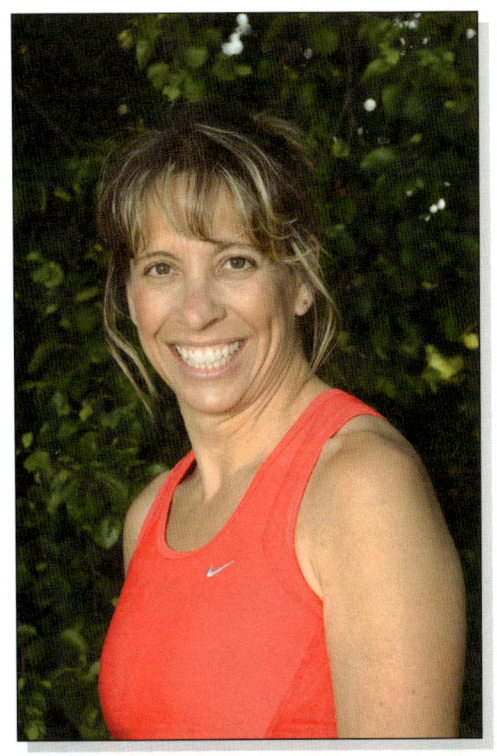

You Can Be Fabulous in Four Weeks

A stronger, more resilient body awaits you. Whether you want to lose weight, sculpt your abs, or take better care of your body, Four Weeks to Fabulous will help you get there.

Learn how to build a stronger body, fuel your body with wholesome foods, improve your overall health, and overcome personal setbacks. This four-week program can be performed in your own home at a time that best works in your schedule.

Is four weeks long enough to promote change and see results? Absolutely. If you follow this plan closely, you will change unhealthy eating habits to healthy ones—and energize your life. Evidence abounds that the amount and type of exercise you will be doing in Four Weeks to Fabulous reduces the risk in adults of early death, coronary heart disease, stroke, high blood pressure, type 2 diabetes, colon and breast cancer, mental decline, and depression. You will feel stronger, more flexible, and even sleep better at night.

Exercise and sound nutrition are without doubt the most important things you can do to invest in your health. Knowing that you are investing in your health, you can expect to spend around thirty dollars for a fitness ball, weights, and a band or tubing—a small investment when you consider the benefits you will receive. Many people have spent that much on vitamins for one month! The truth is, many people have an easier time believing in a pill than the capabilities of their own bodies!

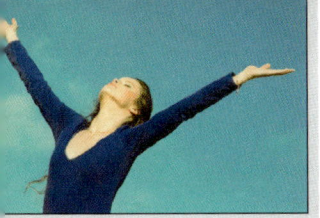

Chapter 1: Success Begins with the Right Attitude

If you have previously struggled to stay with an exercise or diet program, do not skip this chapter. Retraining your brain to think positively toward completing the four-week goal and taking the time to plan around obstacles will bring you to completion and success.

To gain insight into your true purpose and drive behind following the Four Weeks to Fabulous program, answer the following questions:

What are my two main reasons for wanting to follow the Four Weeks to Fabulous program?
1.

2.

What are the two main reasons holding me back from exercising and eating well now?
1.

2.

Four Weeks to Fabulous is a stepping-stone and inspiration on your journey to feeling your best.

1

Four Weeks to Fabulous

Now that you have stated clearly why you want to achieve success and what has been holding you back, create a plan to succeed. For example, if your two reasons for wanting to complete Four Weeks to Fabulous are to lose weight and feel better and the main reasons you have not until now are because of little time and energy, your action plan may be something like this:

I will make time early in the mornings to exercise while I still have energy, and I will shop on Sundays so that I have meals planned for the week.

What is your action plan? Be sure to write it down, and also verbalize it to others. People who verbalize their intentions to others are 80 percent more likely to achieve them.

My action plan is to…

You cannot fail on your wellness journey. There is no finish line.

If you are struggling with creating an action plan, read on for tips on how to plan around the obstacles and excuses.

Plan around the obstacles and excuses.

Making time in your day to exercise, shop, and eat right will be critical to a successful Four Weeks to Fabulous. The exercises, meals, and even the shopping list are laid out and thought out for you. Now all you have to do is look at your schedule closely and make time for exercise and eating well

Chapter 1: Success Begins with the Right Attitude

in your day. Note that this is not the same as finding time in your day, which implies that you have to squeak Four Weeks to Fabulous in your busy schedule, but instead *making* time, which implies that you examine your priorities and identify things that are taking your time that are not moving you in a positive direction, and replacing those things with exercise and eating well.

Here are some questions to help you decide when in the day and week you will be able to best follow the Four Weeks plan. I recommend getting out a calendar to mark out your new plans.

1. What day of the week will be the best day for me to grocery shop for the ingredients in the Four Week plan?

2. What time of day is the most convenient time for me to exercise?

3. What time of day do I enjoy exercising the most?

4. Where do I want to exercise?

5. Will an accountability partner help me achieve my four-week goal?

6. What is my backup plan if my partner bails?

7. What do I foresee as an obstacle (or obstacles) that might keep me from not exercising or eating well?

8. How can I plan around obstacle(s)?

Eating well and being active—even a little every day—is valuable in fostering continuity. Something is always better than nothing.

Four Weeks to Fabulous

Mark on the calendar your completion date and plan to give yourself a non-food reward when you complete the program. Make a big deal out of the last day!

Replace the excuses with positives.

Let your thoughts about exercise and eating healthily always remain positive. If you relate to any of these excuses, try replacing them with the positive thoughts here.

Instead of Saying This Excuse…	Say *This* to Change Your Attitude
I don't enjoy exercise.	I will gradually learn to enjoy being active and approach exercise as a new adventure.
Exercise is boring.	I will experiment with different options to make exercise fun such as music and friends and even new exercise clothing.
Being fat runs in my family.	Action and habits are superior to genetics.
I love food so I don't diet.	I can still eat foods I enjoy in moderation.
I don't have the energy to exercise.	If I don't have energy after 15 minutes into the exercises I can always stop.
Healthy food is too expensive.	Healthy food can be less expensive and will keep me from getting sick and spending money on medications.
I don't like to sweat.	Sweating is the way my skin gets exercise. I will have beautiful, radiant skin when I'm done.
I don't have time to exercise.	Even short bouts of exercise can make a big difference.
I do housework all day so I already exercise.	While I do housework I will intentionally try to get my heart rate high and work my heart and lungs.

Fortunately, attitudes are learned, so we are able to train ourselves to talk with an optimistic voice instead of a pessimistic one. A good attitude is a choice—so choose to be positive today. Don't let what you can't do interfere with what you can do!

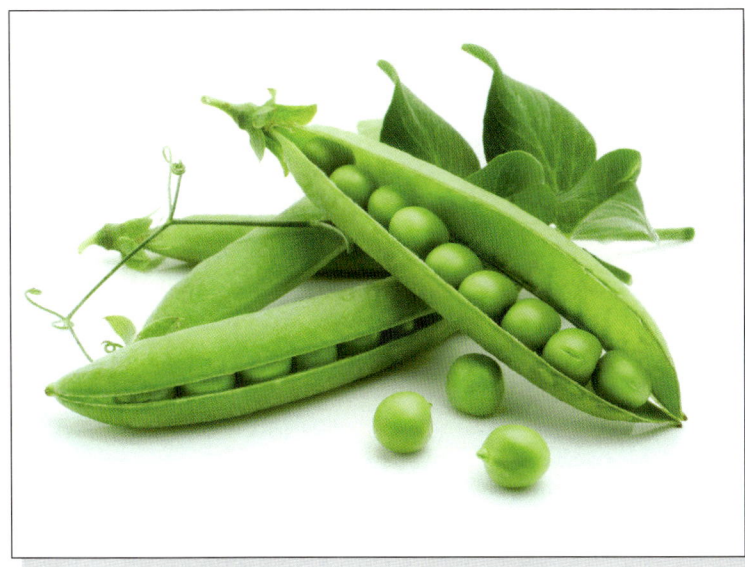

Chapter 2: Four Weeks to Fabulous Nutrition Plan

To accommodate your demanding schedule, the Four Weeks to Fabulous Nutrition Plan offers quick and easy meals and recipes and is designed for busy, health-minded people who desire to:

- Lose weight
- Lower cholesterol
- Control diabetes
- Reduce the risk of cancer
- Increase bone mass
- Improve brain function
- Improve digestive disorders
- Slow the aging process

Four Weeks to Fabulous

With so much health information making the headlines, be reassured that these recipes are based on recommendations from the American Cancer Society, American Heart Association, and American Diabetes Association and are:

- Low in refined sugars and starches
- Low in total fat
- Low in saturated and trans fats
- Low in cholesterol
- Low in sodium
- High in soluble and insoluble fiber
- High in nutrients, minerals, and phytochemicals (anti-cancer compounds)

Begin each day, first thing, with a glass of water to get your digestive system moving and metabolism started. Continue to sip on water throughout the entire day.

The Four Weeks to Fabulous menus are meant to be as satisfying as they are good for you. Follow the daily menus or choose from the compilation of meal choices for breakfast, lunch, dinner, and snacks/desserts. A shopping list is included so that you can be sure you have the ingredients you need!

Quality of food is incredibly important, but so is quantity. Unless you know how many calories to eat, you may still gain weight and overeat. Just how many calories should you consume in a day? You can estimate how many calories you need a day to maintain your current weight by using the following formulas:

Chapter 2: Four Weeks to Fabulous Nutrition Plan

For sedentary people: Weight x 14 = estimated calories/day

For moderately active people: Weight x 17 = estimated calories/day

For active people: Weight x 20 = estimated calories/day

Note: Moderately Active is defined as 3-4 aerobic sessions per week. Active is defined as 5-7 aerobic sessions per week.

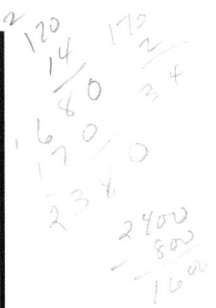

If you desire to lose weight, create a deficit of 400 to 800 calories from your estimated calories/day needed. This deficit should be from both exercise (burning calories) and decreasing caloric intake (eating fewer calories). Rapid weight loss (five pounds or more per week) is rarely maintained, and studies show that a balanced approach to weight loss is the most effective.

In the Four Weeks program, there is a sample menu for each day that contains an average of 1800 calories, of which approximately 21% is protein, 44% is carbohydrate, and 35% is fat. Use this menu to guide and inspire you to eating well, but feel free to use your own favorite healthy recipes. Since every individual's caloric needs are different, you may need to fine-tune your intake to reach your final goal. For example, if you find that you are extremely hungry an hour after dinner, you may want to slightly increase your serving size at dinner the next day. Likewise, if you have not lost weight or inches the first week, you may need to decrease portion sizes.

Refrain from eating after seven p.m. for best weight loss results. Going to bed slightly hungry will burn off pounds.

Four Weeks to Fabulous

Here are some examples of a single serving size, according to the United States Dietary Association:

- Pasta and rice equal to slightly smaller than a tennis ball
- Meat, fish, or poultry the size of a deck of cards
- Snacks, such as pretzels and chips, the size of a cupped handful
- Potato the size of a computer mouse
- Bagel the size of a hockey puck
- Vegetables or fruit about the size of your fist
- Cheese the size of your thumb

Along with the huge effort you are making to reach your goals, make the next step and cut the processed foods out of your food choices. Your goal will be to eat foods that come straight from the source—the earth. Fresh or frozen fruits and vegetables (without salt or sugar added), eggs, milk, cheese, unprocessed meats, whole wheat flour, and honey are all one step away from the earth, not five or six.

Frozen vegetables have the same or increased nutritional value as fresh vegetables and often cost much less. Check to be sure there are no other added ingredients such as salt or sauce.

Chapter 2: Four Weeks to Fabulous Nutrition Plan

Here are some foods that you will want to avoid that are full of preservatives and void of naturally occurring nutrients:

- soda
- anything with refined and enriched white flour
- chips
- fast foods
- processed meats and cheeses
- candy
- prepackaged cookies
- nutrition drinks/shakes unless made with natural ingredients

If you crave sugar, try these tips: keep sweets out of your surroundings, go for a short walk, chew sugar-free gum, drink a glass of lemon water or simply keep sugary food portions small and take the time to enjoy the experience.

Four Weeks to Fabulous

Here are some tips to remember when you go to the store in order to avoid the processed food trap:

- Avoid high-fructose corn syrup (HFCS) and artificially sweetened foods.
- Avoid foods that say "enriched" or "refined."
- If artificial flavors are added—avoid it.
- Try to find the low-salt version—or better yet, the no-salt version.
- Fresh is best.
- Look for products with natural ingredients on the label.

Here's a good rule of thumb: if you can't pronounce a food ingredient, then don't eat it.

Reading labels before you buy will save you calories, cut out preservatives, and enhance your eating experience. Although everyone eats processed foods at times, the more you avoid them, the faster you will see results toward your goal.

About the Four Weeks to Fabulous Menus

Four Weeks recipes can be prepared in thirty minutes or less and have few ingredients. Recipes are based on guidelines from the American Heart Association, American Diabetes Association, and American Dietetic Association and are low-sodium, low-fat, simple gourmet style, and easy to follow. Be sure to use the convenient shopping list for once-a-week stocking up.

If you have special dietetic needs, be sure to consult with your physician, registered dietitian, or certified diabetes educator who can address your individual needs.

You may want to mix and match breakfasts, lunches, dinners, snacks, and desserts according to your tastes if you prefer one option over the other. Enjoy!

Menus

Monday

Breakfast
* 1/3 cup granola with ½ cup low-fat plain yogurt
* ½ cup fresh berries
* 1 cup unsweetened or lightly honey-sweetened coffee or tea

Fab Factoid: One tablespoon of sugar or sucrose contains 46 calories, while one tablespoon of honey has 65 calories. Though honey may have more calories, it is much sweeter so less is used. Honey also has a healthier Glycemic Index (GI), the measure of impact a food has on the blood-glucose levels. The lower the GI rating, the slower the absorption of sugars into the bloodstream. A lower GI allows for a more gradual and healthier digestive process. Honey also has minerals that table sugar lacks.

Midmorning Snack
* 1 sliced apple with 2 tablespoons all-natural peanut butter

Lunch
* Quesadilla: Spread one 100% whole-wheat tortilla with ¼ cup mashed avocado, ¼ cup nonfat refried beans or black beans, and 1/8 cup shredded cheddar cheese. Fold in half and heat quesadilla until cheese melts—either in microwave or on stovetop.
* Baked tortilla chips (12 triangles) with salsa

Midday Snack
* 10 raw or dry-roasted unsalted peanuts, almonds, pecans, walnuts, or pistachios

Four Weeks to Fabulous

Dinner

* **Tilapia:** Drizzle 1 teaspoon olive oil over frozen tilapia fillet and coat fillet sides in a breading made with half Italian breadcrumbs, half Parmesan cheese, and a dash of garlic salt. Place on cookie sheet sprayed with cooking spray and broil for 10 minutes or until fillet is golden brown and well cooked.
* **Couscous:** Directions are on the package. Use plain couscous, not a flavored mix, made with low-sodium chicken broth and a splash of olive oil.

> *Fab Factoid: Couscous can be found in the rice or pasta section of the market. Couscous is made from durum wheat, the main ingredient in good-quality pasta.*

* **Salad:** 1 cup lettuce, ¼ tomato, ¼ red bell pepper, 3 halved Kalamata olives, 1 teaspoon toasted slivered almonds. Drizzle with olive oil and balsamic vinegar.

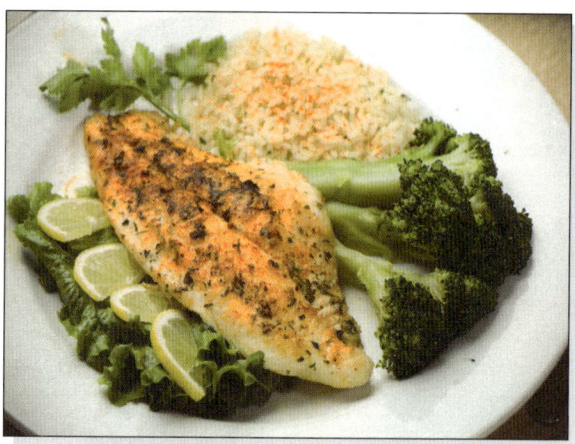

Dessert (optional)

* 1 cup of sugar-free flavored gelatins (any fruit flavor)

Nutrient Analysis for Monday: *1632 calories; 76 g protein; 167 g carbohydrates; 78 g fat; 27 g fiber*

Menus

Tuesday

Breakfast
* 1 cup oatmeal made with nonfat milk served with 1 tablespoon sliced almonds, chopped pecans, or walnuts
* 1/3 cup fresh berries
* 1 poached egg

Midmorning Snack
* 1 banana with 1 tablespoon almond butter

Lunch
* Sesame stir-fry: Cut four asparagus spears into 2-inch pieces and ½ cup tofu into cubes. Cook on medium high in 1 tablespoon sesame oil. Add ¼ cup water and sprinkle with powdered or freshly minced ginger. Add 1 tablespoon low sodium soy sauce and sprinkle with sesame seeds. Stir to coat. Serve with ¾ cup fast-cooking brown rice.

Midday Snack
* 2 cups air-popped popcorn lightly sprinkled with salt
* 1 sliced apple

Dinner
* Chicken strips: Slice a chicken breast into strips. Dip chicken into a bowl with ¼ cup olive oil mixed with a dash of Worcestershire sauce. Dredge in a mixture of half bread crumbs and half Parmesan cheese. Place on a cookie sheet sprayed with nonstick cooking spray.

Four Weeks to Fabulous

    Cook at 425 degrees for 20 minutes, or until chicken is sizzling and golden brown. Serve with ketchup or a little honey.

* Wild rice with toasted slivered almonds: Heat 1 teaspoon olive oil in a medium pot over medium heat. Add 1 cup wild rice, 2 tablespoons sliced almonds, 1 tablespoon minced garlic, 6 sliced green onions, and 1 teaspoon dried thyme. Cook until onions are soft but before garlic is brown. Pour in 2 ½ cups of fat-free low-sodium chicken broth and bring to a boil. Reduce heat to low, cover with a lid, and let cook for 50 minutes or until rice is tender.
* Steamed vegetable (broccoli, asparagus, Brussels sprouts, or green beans—1 cup) or a small salad with 1 tablespoon oil and vinegar dressing.

> *Fab Factoid:* Although both brown rice and wild rice are good for you because they are low in fat, a good source of fiber, and contain the minerals selenium and manganese, wild rice contains slightly less calories per serving.

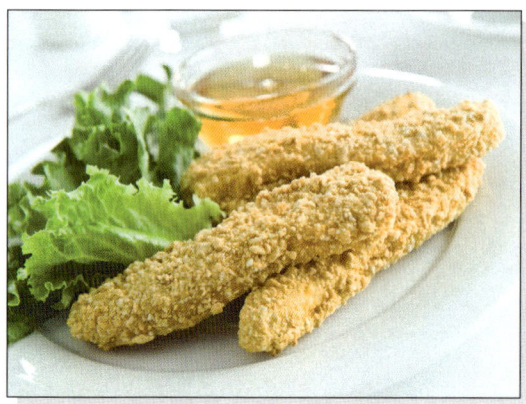

Dessert (Optional)

* ¼ cup fat-free frozen vanilla yogurt with ½ cup sliced strawberries

Nutrient Analysis for Tuesday: *1796 calories, 87 g protein, 210 g carbohydrates, 75 g fat, 30 g fiber*

Menus

Wednesday

Breakfast
* **1 cup shredded wheat cereal, ¾ cup 1% milk, 1 sliced banana, 1 tablespoon slivered almonds**
* **1 to 2 mugs unsweetened or lightly sweetened coffee or tea**

Midmorning Snack
* **Fat-free Greek-style honey yogurt sprinkled with 1 tablespoon granola**

Lunch
* **Salad with chicken: 2 cup salad greens, ¼ cup cucumber, 1/8 cup shredded carrots, 1 slice low sodium deli chicken breast, all drizzled with 1 teaspoon olive oil and sprinkled with balsamic vinegar, toasted nuts and parmesan cheese.**
* **One 100% whole-wheat pita**

Midday Snack
* **1 stick of string cheese**

Dinner
* **Angelhair pasta with shrimp: Sautee in olive oil four sliced green onions, 1 minced garlic clove, 1 tablespoon chopped black olives, and 1 tablespoon sun-dried tomatoes (in olive oil) until onions are soft. Salt and pepper to taste. Add ½ cup of uncooked shrimp and heat until pink. Pour over 1 cup cooked angelhair pasta. Sprinkle with 1 tablespoon shredded Parmesan cheese, if desired.**

Four Weeks to Fabulous

> ***Fab Factoid:*** *Shrimp is low in saturated fat. It is also a good source of niacin, iron, phosphorus, and zinc, and a very good source of protein, vitamin B12, and selenium.*

* **Steamed broccoli**

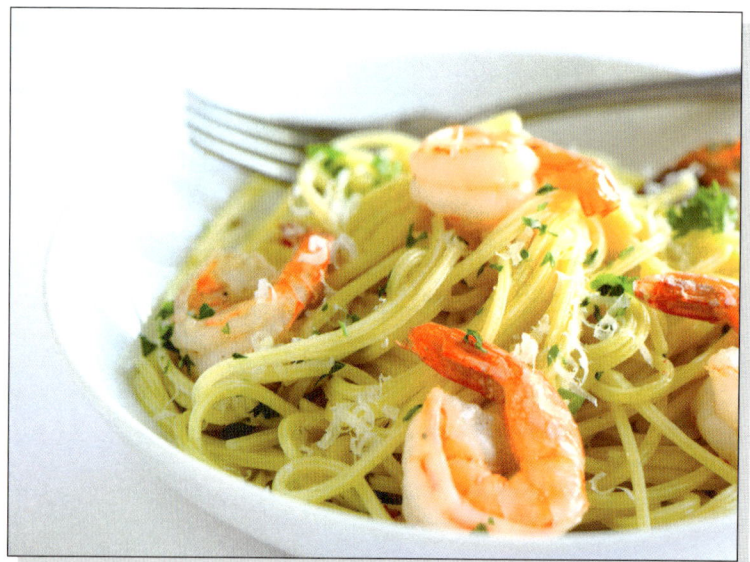

Dessert (optional)
* **Herbal tea such as ginger, lemon, dandelion, or mint tea or sugar-free apple cider hot drink mix**

Nutrient Analysis for Wednesday: *1556 calories, 107 g protein, 190 g carbohydrates, 48 g fat, 22 g fiber*

Menus

Thursday

Breakfast
* ½ 100% whole-wheat bagel spread with 1 tablespoon all-natural peanut butter and 1 teaspoon low-sugar jelly
* 1 pear
* 1 cup 1% milk

Midmorning Snack
* 1 large carrot or 10 baby carrots

Lunch
* Turkey sandwich: 2 slices of 100% whole-wheat bread, 3 ounces thinly sliced lean turkey breast, 1 slice Baby Swiss or Farmer's cheese, 1/4 cup mashed avocado, ½ roasted bell pepper, alfalfa sprouts
* Baked chips (12 chips)

Midday Snack
* Trail mix, ¼ cup

Dinner
* Chili: Fry 1 pound 90% lean hamburger meat (or leaner) sprinkled with 1 tablespoon dried onion flakes, salt, and pepper to taste. Once meat is cooked, drain away fat and then sprinkle with 1 tablespoon chili powder and add 2 cans of low-sodium dark red

Four Weeks to Fabulous

kidney beans (or see tip below) and one 32-ounce can of crushed tomatoes. Simmer over medium-high heat for 30 minutes. Freeze any leftovers for up to 3 months.

> **Fab Cooks Tip:** *To lower the sodium content of canned beans, you can drain and thoroughly rinse them before adding them to recipes. Add a little water back to the recipe to make up for drained liquids.*

* One 100% whole wheat pita

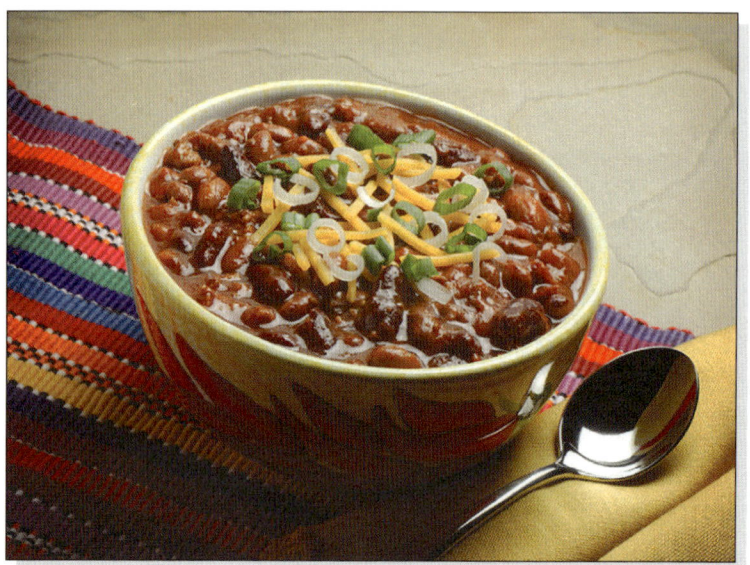

Dessert (optional)
* 4 vanilla wafers with ½ cup light sorbet

Nutrient Analysis for Thursday: *1755 calories, 95 g protein, 238 g carbohydrates, 57 g fat, 33 g fiber*

Menus

Friday

Breakfast
* 1 cup cream of wheat made with skim milk or 1 tablespoon powdered skim milk added after cooking, ½ cup fruit, 8-10 walnuts, ½ teaspoon brown sugar, dash of cinnamon
* 1 to 2 mugs unsweetened or lightly sweetened coffee or tea

Midmorning Snack
* 1 handful of low-fat, reduced sodium wheat crackers and 1/4 cup hummus or 1 string cheese stick

> *Fab Cook's Tip:* Hummus can be made by processing 2 (15-ounce) cans drained and rinsed chickpeas, ½ cup warm water, 3 tablespoons lemon or lime juice, 1 tablespoon tahini (ground sesame paste), 1½ teaspoons ground cumin, 1 tablespoon minced garlic, 1 teaspoon salt, and 2 tablespoons chopped fresh cilantro. Add water if needed. Hummus will keep for several days refrigerated. Tahini can be found next to the peanut butter in the market, or made with 1 cup sesame seeds and 1/3 cup olive oil, processed into a paste.

Lunch
* Chili (1 ½ cups) with 5 low-sodium saltine crackers
* Tangerine

Midday Snack
* 2 cups air-popped popcorn lightly sprinkled with salt

Four Weeks to Fabulous

Dinner

* **Broiled salmon:** Coat a salmon filet with 2 tablespoons sesame oil and 2 tablespoons soy sauce, juice from one lemon, and ½ teaspoon ground ginger. Place salmon on a broiling pan sprayed with nonstick spray and broil for 10-15 minutes or until done. Watch closely.
* **Brown rice pilaf:** Melt 1 tablespoon butter in a pot and add one bunch of chopped green onion or chives (about 6 stalks). Cook until soft. Add 1 cup brown rice and coat rice with butter. Add 2 cups low-sodium chicken broth and 1 tablespoon dried parsley. Stir, then bring to a boil over high heat. After broth comes to a boil, turn heat to low and let broth come to a low boil. Cover with lid and let cook for 40-50 minutes.
* **Fruit salad:** 1 diced apple, 1 sliced banana, one 10-ounce can low-sugar mandarin oranges. Sprinkle with cinnamon and mix together.
* **Steamed green beans**

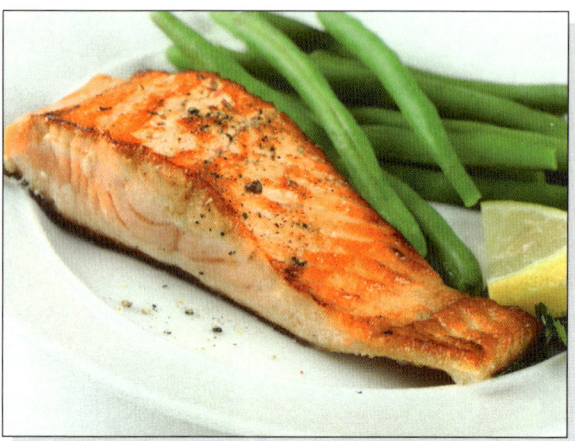

Dessert (optional)

* 1 ounce high cocoa chocolate (60% or more cocoa)

Nutrient Analysis for Friday: *1756 calories, 95 g protein, 212 g carbohydrates, 76 g fat, 31 g fiber*

Menus

Saturday

Breakfast
* **Scrambled veggie eggs:** Sautee 1 tablespoon green onion and ½ finally chopped red or orange bell pepper in 1 teaspoon olive oil. Cook until tender, then add 1 whole egg 1 egg white and mix together.
* **1 piece of 100% whole-wheat toast, spread with 1 tablespoon light (low-sugar) preserves**
* **1 cup grapes**
* **1 to 2 mugs unsweetened or lightly sweetened coffee or tea**

Midmorning Snack
* **1 medium low-fat oatmeal cookie or small low-fat bran or small whole wheat muffin**

Lunch
* **Deli wrap:** Roll one large 100% whole-wheat tortilla around 4 ounces thinly sliced low-sodium deli turkey breast (or other lean lunch meat), ¼ cup sprouts or lettuce, ¼ cup chopped tomato, and ¼ cup mashed avocado. Slice into quarters.

> *Fab Factoid:* Avocados are a fruit, not a vegetable. They contain over twenty essential nutrients, are a great source of vitamin K and folate, and high in heart-healthy mono- and polyunsaturated fats.

* **Baked chips (12)**

Four Weeks to Fabulous

Midday Snack
* Celery stalks (unlimited) with 2 tablespoons natural peanut or almond butter

Dinner
* Meat patty: Mix 1 pound 90% lean ground beef (or leaner) with one egg, 2 tablespoons Italian bread crumbs, 1 teaspoon flaked dried onions, 1 teaspoon dried parsley, salt and pepper. Form into a patty and fry in a skillet sprayed with nonstick cooking spray. Cook on medium heat until desired doneness. Drain fat.
* Baby red potatoes: diced and sautéed in olive oil, salt, pepper, and fresh parsley (1 cup)
* Roasted asparagus (4 spears): Spray a cooking sheet and asparagus with nonstick cooking spray. Spray asparagus with cooking spray. Sprinkle asparagus with sea salt, pepper, and a few sprinkles of balsamic vinegar. Broil 5 minutes or until asparagus is tender.

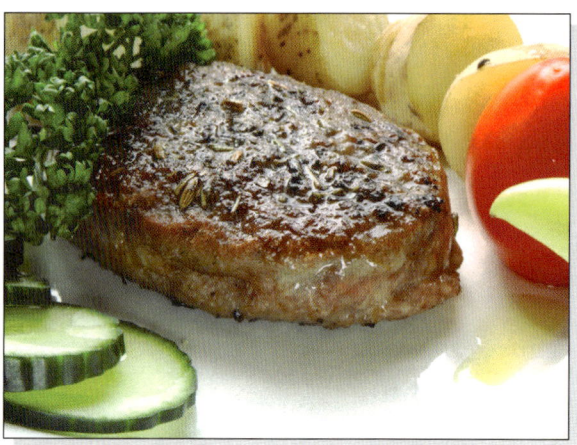

Dessert (optional)
* 15 chocolate-covered raisins, blueberries, or cherries

Nutrient Analysis for Saturday: *1789 calories, 83 g protein, 201 g carbohydrates, 73 g fat, 30 g fiber*

Menus

Sunday

Breakfast
* One 100% whole wheat English muffin with 1 thin slice low fat cheese
* 1 fried egg in olive oil
* 1 kiwi fruit
* 1 to 2 mugs unsweetened or lightly honey-sweetened coffee or tea

> *Fab Factoid:* Don't be afraid to eat eggs—they are a good source of protein, riboflavin, vitamin B12, and phosphorus, and a very good source of selenium. Eggs also contain 210 mg of cholesterol—up to almost your entire allowance of cholesterol for the day which is 300 mg or less. Still, eggs are fine to eat up to four yolks a week.

Midmorning Snack
* 2 graham crackers with a small glass of 1% milk

Lunch
* Greek salad: Chop 1 tomato, ½ bell pepper, and ½ cucumber and mix with 1 cup spinach in a bowl with crumbled reduced-fat feta cheese. Drizzle with 2 teaspoons olive oil and 2 tablespoon red wine or balsamic vinegar.
* One 100% whole-wheat pita

Four Weeks to Fabulous

Midday Snack
* 1 6-ounce container of low-fat cottage cheese (optional: sprinkled with slivered almonds and 1/2 cup berries)

Dinner
* Pesto pasta with chicken: Cook penne noodles until done. Mix with jarred pesto or make your own. Pesto: blend a cup of basil leaves (fresh spinach can be used for a milder flavor), ¼ cup toasted nuts (pine nuts are best, but any kind works except peanuts), ¼ cup olive oil, and ¼ cup parmesan cheese, and two cloves of garlic. Add salt to taste.
* Chicken: Cut a small chicken breast into thin strips and sauté in a small amount of olive oil. Add salt and pepper taste. Serve on top of pasta.
* Sautéed spinach in a small amount of olive oil, minced garlic, pine nuts, salt and pepper

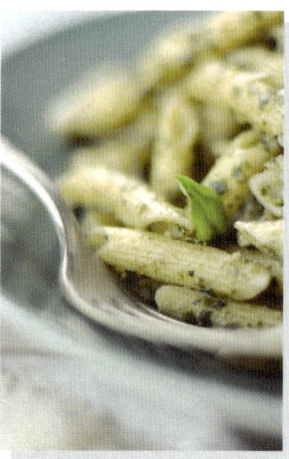

Dessert (optional)
* 1 frozen fruit bar or ¼ cup mixed fruit

Nutrient Analysis for Wednesday: *1640 calories, 88 g protein, 203 g carbohydrates, 61 g fat, 29 g fiber*

Breakfast Options

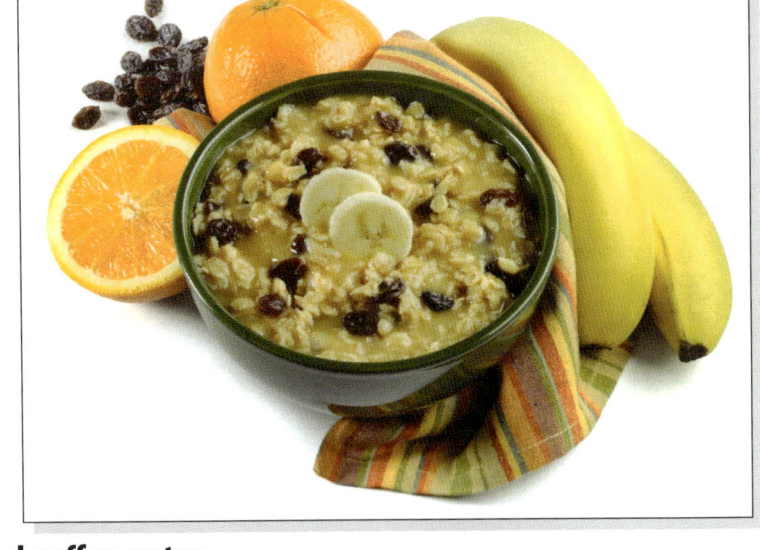

For recipes, see the corresponding menu for that day of the week.

Choice 1 Monday
1/3 cup granola
½ cup low-fat plain yogurt
½ cup fresh berries
1 cup unsweetened or lightly sweetened coffee or tea

Choice 2 Tuesday
1 cup oatmeal made with nonfat milk (½ old fashioned oats, 1 cup milk)
5 almonds, pecans, or walnuts
1/3 cup fresh berries
1 poached egg

Choice 3 Wednesday
1 cup shredded wheat, 3/4 cup 1% milk, 1 sliced banana, and 1 tablespoon slivered almonds
1 to 2 mugs unsweetened or lightly sweetened coffee or tea

Four Weeks to Fabulous

Choice 4 Thursday
1/2 100% whole-wheat bagel, 1 tablespoon all-natural peanut butter, 1 teaspoon low-sugar jelly
1 pear
1 cup 1% milk

Choice 5 Friday
1 cup cream of wheat or rice made with skim milk, 1/2 cup fruit, 8-10 walnuts, ½ teaspoon brown sugar, dash of cinnamon
1 to 2 mugs unsweetened or lightly sweetened coffee or tea

Choice 6 Saturday
Scrambled veggie eggs
1 piece of 100% whole-wheat toast, spread with 1 tablespoon light preserves
1 cup grapes
1 to 2 mugs unsweetened or lightly sweetened coffee or tea

Choice 7 Sunday
One 100% whole wheat English muffin (toasted, no butter) with 1 thin slice low-fat cheese
1 fried egg in olive oil
1 kiwi fruit
1 to 2 mugs unsweetened or lightly sweetened coffee or tea

Lunch Options

Lunch Options

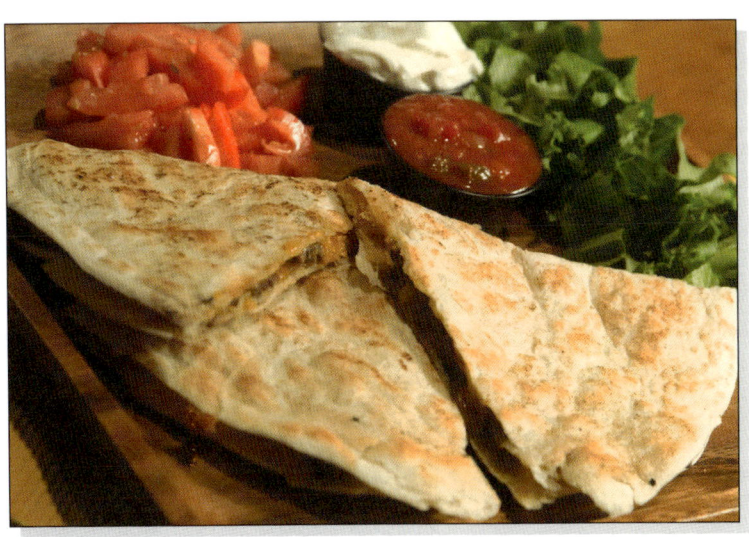

For recipes, see the corresponding menu for that day of the week.

Choice 1 Monday
Quesadilla
Baked tortilla chips (12 triangles), with salsa if desired

Choice 2 Tuesday
Sesame stir-fry
Fast-cooking brown rice

Choice 3 Wednesday
Salad with chicken
One 100% whole-wheat pita

Choice 4 Thursday
Turkey sandwich
Baked chips (12 chips)

Choice 5 Friday
Chili (1½ cups) with 5 low-sodium saltine crackers
Tangerine

Choice 6 Saturday
Deli wrap
Baked chips (12)

Choice 7 Sunday
Greek salad
One 100% whole-wheat pita

Four Weeks to Fabulous

Dinner Options

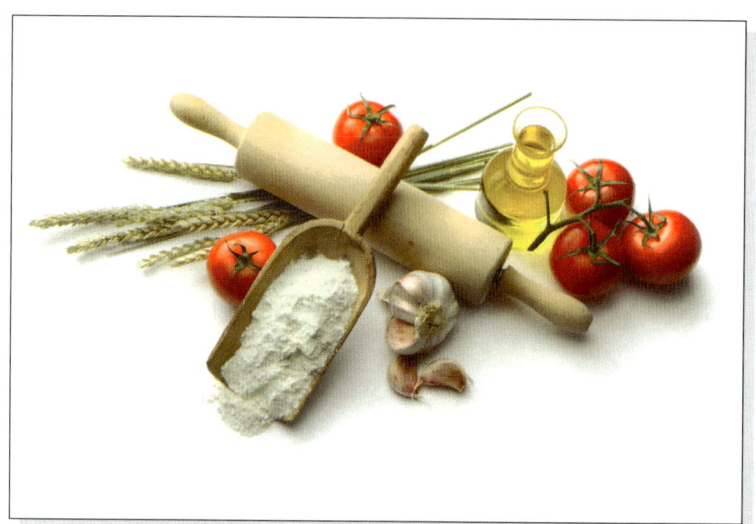

For recipes, see the corresponding menu for that day of the week.

Choice 1 Monday
Baked tilapia
Couscous
Colorful salad

Choice 2 Tuesday
Chicken strips
Wild rice with toasted almonds
Steamed vegetable (broccoli, asparagus, Brussels sprouts, or green beans or a small salad)

Choice 3 Wednesday
Angelhair pasta with shrimp
Steamed broccoli

Choice 4 Thursday
Chili
One 100% whole wheat pita

Choice 5 Friday
Broiled salmon
Brown rice pilaf
Fruit salad
Steamed green beans

Choice 6 Saturday
Meat patty
Sautéed baby red potatoes
Roasted asparagus

Choice 7 Sunday
Pesto pasta
Sautéed chicken
Sautéed spinach

Snacks

- 2 cups air-popped popcorn lightly sprinkled with salt
- 1/2 fat-free vanilla yogurt sprinkled with granola
- 1 small tangerine
- 1 low-fat mozzarella cheese stick
- 1 large carrot or 10 baby carrots
- ½ cup trail mix
- 1 sugar-free frozen fruit bar
- 1 12-ounce skim milk latte
- 5 whole-wheat crackers with baby Swiss cheese
- Celery stalks (unlimited) with 2 tablespoons natural peanut or almond butter
- 1 sliced apple with 2 tablespoons natural peanut or almond butter
- 1 small banana with 2 tablespoons natural peanut or almond butter
- 10 raw or dry-roasted almonds, pecans, walnuts, or pistachios
- 1 banana with one-inch square of high cocoa chocolate (65% or more cocoa)
- 1 handful of wheat crackers and 1/4 cup hummus
- 1 Kashi® TLC® chewy bar
- 1 hard-boiled egg
- 1 6-ounce container of low-fat cottage cheese (optional: sprinkle with slivered almonds and 1/2 cup berries)
- 1 fruit of any kind
- 2 graham crackers with a small glass of nonfat milk
- 1 cup of pretzels
- 1 medium low-fat oatmeal cookie or bran muffin

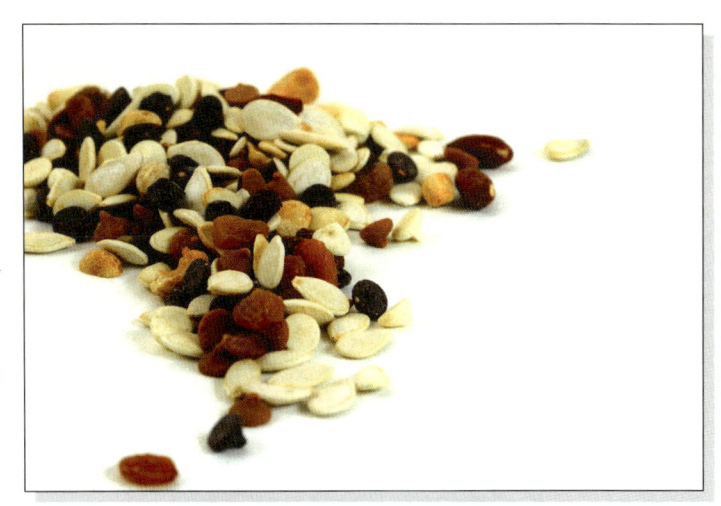

Four Weeks to Fabulous

Desserts

- Fresh berries and vanilla yogurt
- Honeydew, cantaloupe, and watermelon
- Plum, peach, apricot or nectarine
- Pineapple
- 1 fruit popsicle
- 1 cup sugar-free gelatin
- 1 cup sugar free cider, diet hot chocolate, or hot tea
- 1 ounce of high cocoa chocolate (60% or more cocoa)
- 1 small piece maple candy
- 3 medium meringues
- 15 dark chocolate-covered raisins, blueberries, or cherries
- 1 small mint patty
- Vanilla Wafers with 1/2 cup light sorbet
- 1/2 cup fat-free frozen vanilla yogurt with 1/4 cup sliced strawberries

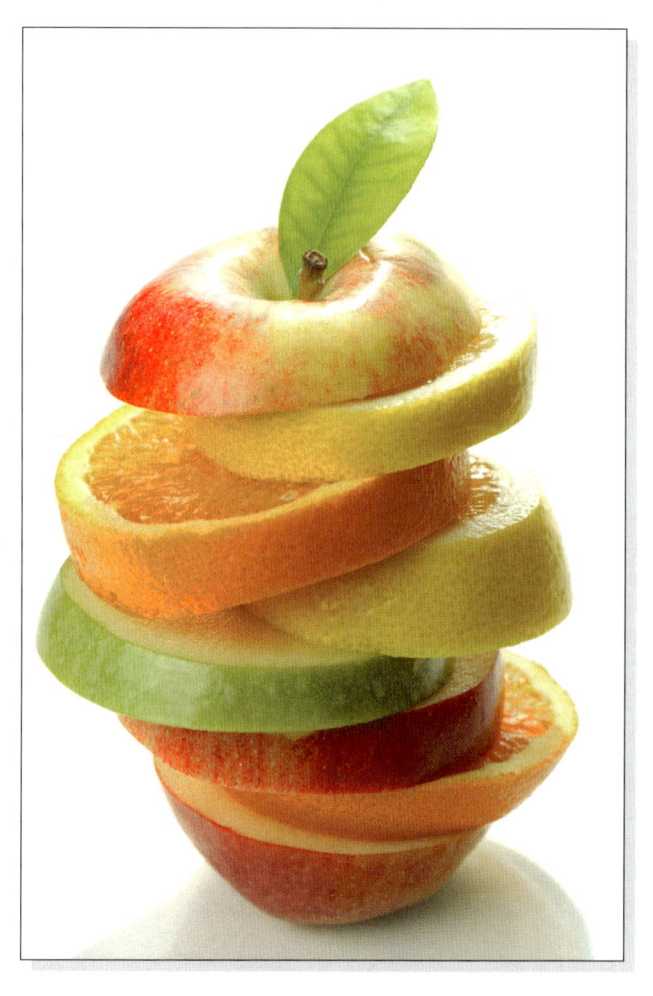

Shopping List

Make shopping easy by using this Four Weeks to Fabulous shopping list. While you're in the cupboard, throw away any foods that may tempt you take a detour from the Four Weeks to Fabulous menu.

Beverages
- ☐ Coffee or tea
- ☐ Sugar-free cider drink mix

Breads
- ☐ Bagels, 100% whole-wheat
- ☐ Bread, 100% whole-wheat
- ☐ English muffin, 100% whole-wheat
- ☐ Muffin, small bran or whole-wheat
- ☐ Oatmeal cookie, small
- ☐ Pita bread, 100% whole-wheat
- ☐ Tortillas, 100% whole-wheat

Canned Goods
- ☐ Bell pepper, roasted
- ☐ Black beans
- ☐ Black olives
- ☐ Chick peas
- ☐ Chicken broth, low-sodium, fat-free
- ☐ Kalamata olives
- ☐ Mandarin oranges, low-sugar
- ☐ Refried beans, non-fat
- ☐ Red kidney beans, low-sodium
- ☐ Sundried tomatoes in oil
- ☐ Tomatoes, crushed, 32-ounces

Cereals
- ☐ Cream of wheat
- ☐ Granola
- ☐ Shredded wheat
- ☐ Old-fashioned oatmeal

Dry Goods
- ☐ Brown sugar
- ☐ Couscous
- ☐ Cooking spray
- ☐ Italian bread crumbs
- ☐ Pasta (bowtie, angel hair, fettuccine)
- ☐ Powdered skim milk
- ☐ Rice, basmati and wild
- ☐ Quick cooking brown rice

Eggs & Dairy
- ☐ Butter
- ☐ Cheddar cheese, shredded, 2% milk
- ☐ Cheese, Baby Swiss and/or Farmer's
- ☐ Cottage cheese, low-fat
- ☐ Eggs
- ☐ Feta cheese, reduced-fat
- ☐ Milk, Skim and/or 1%
- ☐ Parmesan cheese
- ☐ String cheese, low-fat
- ☐ Tofu, firm
- ☐ Yogurt, non-fat Greek style, honey flavor
- ☐ Yogurt, plain low-fat

Frozen Foods
- ☐ Frozen fruit bar
- ☐ Sorbet, low-sugar
- ☐ Stir-fry vegetables
- ☐ Vanilla yogurt, fat-free, low-sugar

Four Weeks to Fabulous

Fruits & Vegetables
- [ ] Apples
- [ ] Alfalfa or clover sprouts
- [ ] Asparagus
- [ ] Avocado
- [ ] Banana
- [ ] Bell peppers, red, green or orange
- [ ] Berries, fresh or frozen with no sugar added
- [ ] Broccoli
- [ ] Brussel sprouts
- [ ] Carrots
- [ ] Celery
- [ ] Cucumber
- [ ] Garlic
- [ ] Ginger
- [ ] Grapes
- [ ] Green beans
- [ ] Green onions or chives
- [ ] Kiwi
- [ ] Lemon
- [ ] Melon, honeydew, cantaloupe and/or watermelon
- [ ] Onion
- [ ] Parsley
- [ ] Pears
- [ ] Plums, peaches, apricots, pineapple
- [ ] Potatoes, baby red
- [ ] Salad greens (red lettuce, spinach)
- [ ] Tangerines, nectarines, oranges
- [ ] Tomatoes

Peanut Butter & Nuts
- [ ] Almond butter
- [ ] Peanut butter, all-natural (without added sugar, salt, or vegetable oil)
- [ ] Nuts, peanuts, pine nuts, cashews, pistachios, walnuts, pecans, almonds, raw or dry roasted, unsalted, chopped, sliced or whole
- [ ] Sesame seeds, toasted
- [ ] Tahini

Poultry * Beef * Pork
- [ ] Chicken breast
- [ ] Hamburger meat, 90% lean
- [ ] Roast beef, low-sodium, lean, sliced
- [ ] Turkey breast, low-sodium, sliced

Seafood
- [ ] Salmon, wild caught
- [ ] Shrimp
- [ ] Tilapia

Shopping List

Snacks
- ☐ Baked tortilla chips
- ☐ Chocolate, 60% or more cocoa
- ☐ Chocolate mint patty, small
- ☐ **Dark chocolate-covered raisins, blueberries, or cherries**
- ☐ Gelatin, sugar free, fruit-flavored
- ☐ Graham crackers, low-fat
- ☐ Hummus
- ☐ Kashi bar
- ☐ Popcorn
- ☐ Pretzels
- ☐ Saltine crackers, low-sodium
- ☐ Trail mix
- ☐ Vanilla wafers
- ☐ Wheat crackers, low-sodium

Spices and Condiments
- ☐ Balsamic vinegar
- ☐ Jelly, low-sugar
- ☐ Cinnamon
- ☐ Chili powder
- ☐ Dried parsley
- ☐ Dried onion flakes
- ☐ Garlic salt
- ☐ Ground ginger
- ☐ Honey
- ☐ Ketchup
- ☐ Maple syrup
- ☐ Old and vinegar dressing
- ☐ Olive oil
- ☐ Salsa
- ☐ Salt
- ☐ Soy sauce. low sodium
- ☐ Toasted sesame oil
- ☐ Worcestershire sauce

Other: _____
_____
_____
_____
_____
_____

Chapter 3: Four Weeks to Fabulous Physical Activity Plan

Whatever your goal is—to lose weight, get healthier, or to just feel better—exercise is a critical component. Our bodies were made to move, and the more you move, the better you feel. With just thirty to sixty minutes of activity a day, you will experience strength, energy, and vitality.

This program accommodates two fitness levels: beginner or intermediate. I encourage you to find a fitness level that fits your current fitness status. You may be tempted to jump into the intermediate level without assessing your current fitness level, which you are welcome to do. However, if you become too exhausted or frustrated with the time commitment, you can always move back to the beginner level. The important thing to remember is this—continue the program through week four, whatever level you choose, and don't give up. Starting at the appropriate level, however, will increase your chance of successful completion of the program, and will allow you to achieve the greatest results.

Beginner: If you haven't exercised regularly for a while but are somewhat active, the beginner program would be a good place to begin. As with any exercise program, be sure to check with your physician before starting. If you are not active at all, I encourage you to begin with the Start Walking Program, found in this chapter, until you reach Week 4, at which time you can begin the Four Weeks to Fabulous beginner exercise program. I also

Having a partner join you in your four-week plan makes exercising fun, holds you accountable, and greatly increases your chance of success.

Four Weeks to Fabulous

encourage you to feel free to start the nutritional portion of the program immediately with the Start Walking Program.

Intermediate: If you've been exercising fairly consistently (three times a week for at least two months), you can either start with the Beginner routine or go for the Intermediate workout, which requires more endurance and strength but will also give you greater and quicker results.

Once you have completed the Four Weeks to Fabulous program, you will be ready to move onto Four Weeks to Fantastic and then Four Weeks to Famous programs—the next two books in this three-book series. These programs will bring you to your peak performance and health.

To fully visualize the improvements in your fitness level, I highly recommend that you discover your base fitness level prior to starting. Use the simple fitness tests included in this chapter to assess your cardiovascular fitness and upper body strength. Re-test after four weeks to see improvements.

Chapter 3: Four Weeks to Fabulous Physical Activity Plan

The Starting Line—How Fit Are You?

Find your basic fitness level before embarking on the Four Weeks to Fabulous program. Perform these two fitness tests to assess your cardiovascular fitness and muscular strength. Re-test after four weeks, and you will be pleasantly surprised to see improvements! This is a great way to stay encouraged and motivated and to see positive results—on paper and on you!

Before you begin, get your doctor's approval so your doctor can discuss with you whether it is all right for you to exercise and what can be gained from exercise.

Step Test

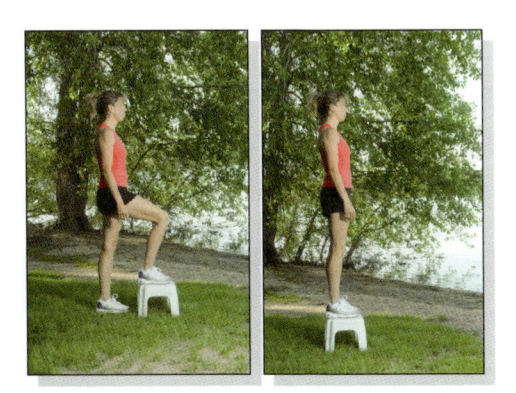

Warm up with a five-minute walk. Find a step about twelve inches high (the bottom stair of a staircase works fine, too), and time yourself going up and down that step at a medium and steady pace for exactly three minutes. At the end of three minutes, sit down and find your pulse at your wrist or neck and count beats for one minute.

Four Weeks to Fabulous

Mark your results here, along with the date you took the test.

Before Four Weeks: Date:_____ Heart Rate: _____
After Four Weeks: Date:_____ Heart Rate: _____

If you are a man and count over 100 heartbeats, or are a woman and count 110 or more heartbeats you could use some aerobic conditioning.

Push-Ups

Warm up with a five-minute walk, and include stretching and moving your arms. Perform a proper push-up by placing hands on the ground even with your chest and just under the shoulders. Keep your body straight without raising your rear end. Count how many push-ups you can do in one minute. It's OK if you can't continue for a full minute. Record how many you can do until complete exhaustion. Record your results here, along with the date you perform the test.

Before Four Weeks: Date:_____ # Push-ups: _____
After Four Weeks: Date:_____ # Push-ups: _____

If you are unable to do a standard push-up at all, don't be discouraged! The Four Weeks Strength Training program is here to help you to increase your upper body strength.

If you are a man and performed fifteen or fewer properly executed push-ups, or are a woman and performed ten or fewer push-ups, you will benefit greatly from the Four Weeks to Fabulous Strength Training program and should see significant improvements in just four weeks. Test after four weeks and record above.

Chapter 3: Four Weeks to Fabulous Physical Activity Plan

Start Walking—Achieving Base Fitness Before Beginning Four Weeks Physical Activity Plan

Walking is one of the easiest ways to exercise. You can do it almost anywhere and at any time, and it is also inexpensive; all you need are comfortable shoes and clothing. Use this walking program three to five times a week to achieve base fitness before you begin the Four Weeks to Fabulous routine.

	Warm up Time	Fast Walk Time*	Cool Down Time	Total Time
Week 1	Walk slowly 5 min	Walk briskly 5 min	Walk slowly 5 min	15 min
Week 2	Walk slowly 5 min	Walk briskly 8 min	Walk slowly 5 min	19 min
Week 3	Walk slowly 5 min	Walk briskly 11 min	Walk slowly 5 min	23 min
Week 4	Walk slowly 5 min	Walk briskly 14 min	Walk slowly 5 min	27 min

Four Weeks to Fabulous

Five-Minute Stretch Routine—Before and After Walking

Hold each stretch at just the point of slight discomfort, but not pain, for a count of ten. Use a support for balance, if necessary. Feel free to repeat the stretch routine.

Hamstring Stretch

1. Take a small step forward with your left foot, straighten your left leg, and bend your right knee slightly.

2. Lift the toes up on your left foot and lean forward, keeping your back flat and chest forward. You will feel the stretch in your back and the back of your left thigh. For a greater stretch, lift toes up more.

3. Hold for a count of ten, then switch legs.

Calf and Hip Stretch

1. Take a giant step forward with your left foot.

2. Bend your left knee so your shin is vertical but your knee is not extending beyond your toes. Keep your right heel on the ground and your right leg straight behind you.

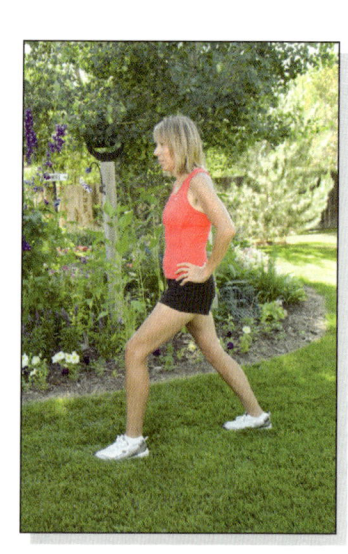

Chapter 3: Four Weeks to Fabulous Physical Activity Plan

3. Stand tall, extending the top of your head to the sky and keeping your stomach muscles tight. Try not to arch your back. You will feel the stretch in your right calf and hip.

4. Hold for a count of ten, then switch legs.

Quad Stretch

1. Stand tall, bend your right leg at the knee behind you, and grasp your right toes with your right hand, keeping your right knee pointed toward the ground.

2. Pull gently to stretch the front of thigh, hip, and shin. Tilt the pelvis forward and keep both knees together for the greatest stretch.

Shoulder and Back Stretch

1. Stand tall, raise your right arm up toward the sky.

2. Bend your right elbow so your hand is behind your head.

3. Grasp your right elbow with your left hand, and gently pull to the left.

4. Hold for a count of ten, then release.

5. Switch arms and repeat.

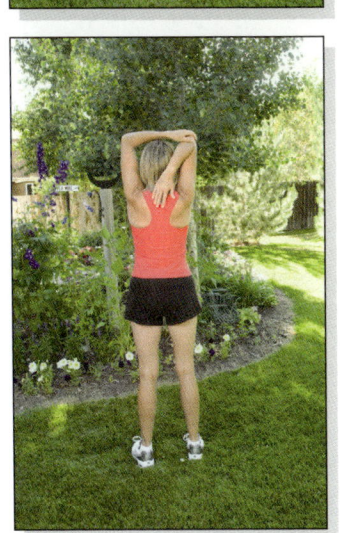

Four Weeks to Fabulous

Let's begin! Once you are ready to begin, your workout each week will consist of two components: Endurance and Strength Training.

Workout Schedule

Day	Activity
Monday	Endurance and Strength
Tuesday	Endurance
Wednesday	Endurance and Strength
Thursday	Endurance
Friday	Endurance and Strength
Saturday	Endurance
Sunday	Rest

Endurance

At first the sound of the word *endurance* may be intimidating, but it simply means strengthening the heart and lungs. The Four Weeks to Fabulous endurance program starts simply with brisk walking every day, but you can use any cardio machine (treadmill, stationary bicycle, stair climber, or elliptical machine) or bicycle, swim, cross-country ski, or do any other aerobic activity in place of walking. Cardio fitness classes—such as spinning, dancing, or aerobics—can also be done in place of your endurance workouts. The intent is to get your heart rate high enough to cause your heart and lungs to get stronger, while also burning away fat. Be sure to do the stretches found in the Start Walking Program before and after your endurance workouts.

To give you an opportunity to increase cardiovascular fitness and even burn more calories, try the twenty-minute interval workout at the end of this chapter that can be done in addition to or included as a part of the

Make it fun—if you don't want to walk, find an activity that you find more enjoyable.

Chapter 3: Four Weeks to Fabulous Physical Activity Plan

endurance workout. Do not do the interval training workout two days in a row. Interval training is intense and without rest can increase your risk of injury.

Strength Training

The Four Weeks to Fabulous program contains three days a week of a strength training circuit that is performed with no rest time between exercises. Because of this, you will be breathing hard and working the cardiovascular system which will boost caloric expenditure. Because there is no rest time, I highly recommend that you read through the exercises first and make the equipment readily available.

Following the order of exercises is important. By the end of the set you should feel the muscles fatigue and slightly burn. If you do not feel slight discomfort, increase the resistance or weights used.

To add further difficulty, try increasing the repetitions and slowing down the movement. Although the first week the strength training routine may only take around fifteen minutes, weeks 2 through 4 kick it up a notch and will take more time because circuits are repeated.

Warm up for at least five minutes by first walking for a few minutes, then march and add light jumping. Add arms and do some jumping jacks or jump roping. You can also use your endurance workout for the day as your warm-up for the strength training portion.

If you feel fatigued before beginning your workout, don't bail but instead start with lighter resistance and repetitions. You may surprise yourself and end up having an awesome workout.

Always give your body one day in between strength training workouts to recover and avoid injury.

Weight-lifting or cycling gloves are recommended—they protect your hands and increase your grip.

Don't hold your breath when strength training; breathe throughout the movement.

Four Weeks to Fabulous

If the exercise becomes too easy, advance to a tube with heavier resistance.

For the strength-training workout, you will need the following equipment:

- A five-pound pair of dumbbells, possibly eight and ten as needed with strength gain
- Gliders (large furniture movers, hard plastic Frisbees, or even disposable Styrofoam plates also work well, although they may need replaced often)
- Resistance bands, light or medium to start, and heavy as needed with strength gain, and door jam holder
- A 55-cm fitness ball if you are 5'0" to 5'6" tall or a 65-cm ball if you are 5'7" to 6'1" tall (a larger ball may be needed if you have long legs for your height or have back problems)

The fitness ball will be very firm when properly inflated. Thighs should be close to parallel to the floor when sitting on the ball, although it is acceptable if your hips are slightly higher than your knees.

Gliders, light, medium and heavy bands, weight and balls are available for purchase separately or as a package at www.2bfit.net.

Now, get started and be ready for a fabulous transformation!

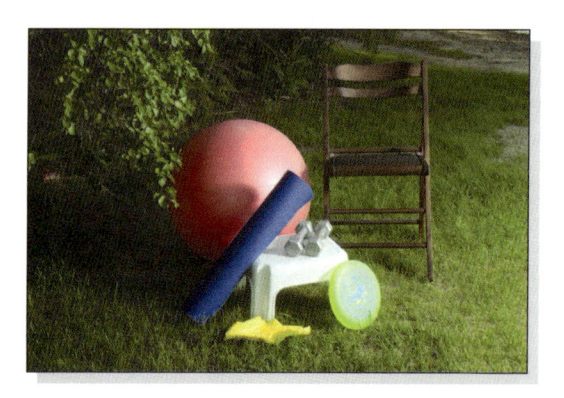

Chapter 3: Four Weeks to Fabulous Physical Activity Plan

Four Week Exercise Descriptions

Chair Squat

Stand with your feet shoulder-width apart. Keeping your back straight, bend from your knees and hips and lower yourself down to a sitting position. Stop just before your hips contact the chair, holding squat for two seconds before returning to starting position.

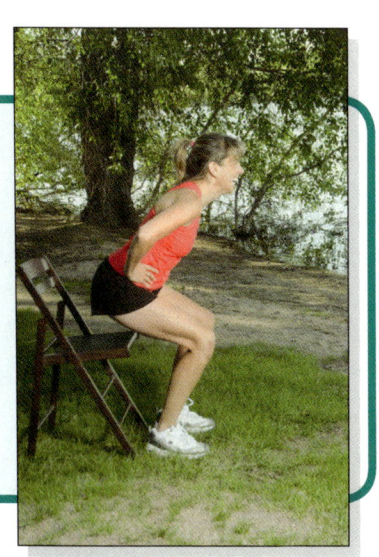

Band Rows
(Palms Down progressing to Palms Up & Palms In)

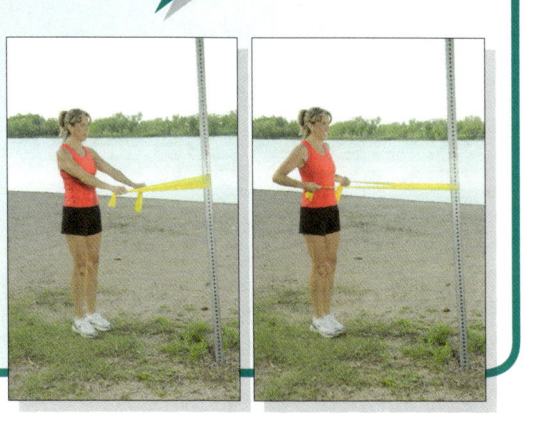

Wrap band around a sturdy object in front of you with arms extended in front of you until you feel good resistance from the band. With palms down and keeping body tall, slowly bend elbows pulling band toward yourself in a rowing motion while keeping arms close to body. Keep your shoulders relaxed, squeezing shoulder blades together. (On subsequent weeks when instructed to turn palms up or in, rotate your hands.)

Four Weeks to Fabulous

Four Week Exercise Descriptions

Dumbbell Hammer Curl to Shoulder Press

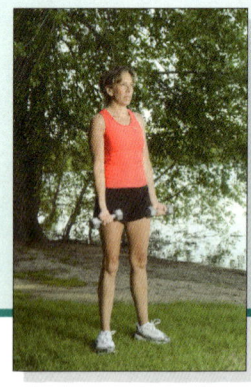

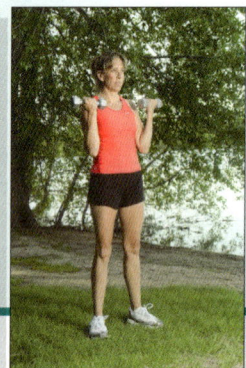

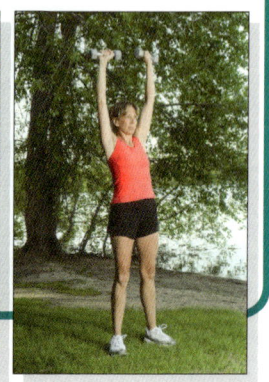

Stand with weights in hands, arms hanging at your sides, palms facing each other. Bend your elbows, curling the weights to your shoulders, and press both weights directly overhead. Lower weights back down to shoulders then down to your sides.

Side Plank on Elbow

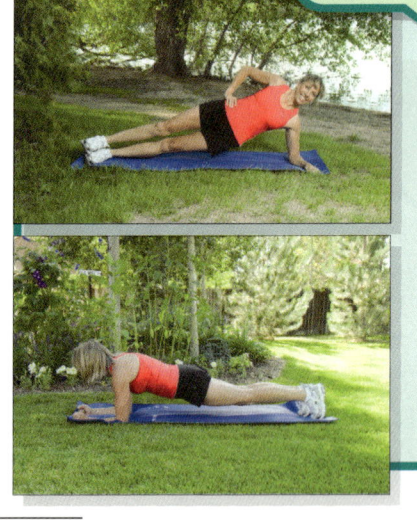

Lie on your side with your legs straight. Prop yourself up with your left forearm so your body forms a diagonal line, and put your right hand on your hip. Inhale, brace your abs, and lift your hips. Hold for thirty seconds and maintain steady breathing. If you can't make thirty seconds, hold for five to ten seconds and rest for five until you've completed thirty seconds in the lifted position. Repeat on other side. In later weeks when the exercise has you moving from a side plank to down plank, position your body facedown balanced on your elbows and toes with your back flat.

Chapter 3: Four Weeks to Fabulous Physical Activity Plan

Four Week Exercise Descriptions

Band Bicep Curls

Holding a grip in each hand, stand on the band with both feet. Palms facing forward, elbows into your sides, bend elbows curling your hands up to your shoulders then slowly return to starting position.

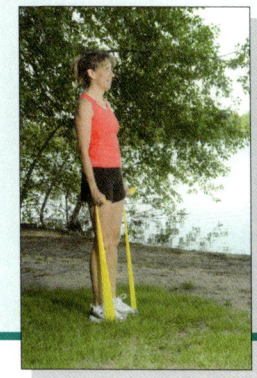

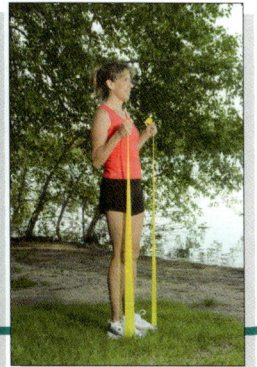

Reverse Crunch

Start by lying on your back, legs extended up toward the ceiling, hands under your hips. Head and shoulders are rolled up off the floor to hold an abdominal contraction. Slowly lower both legs toward the floor, making sure to keep your low back in contact with the floor. Hold legs above the floor for three to five seconds then return to start. Straighten legs for an additional challenge.

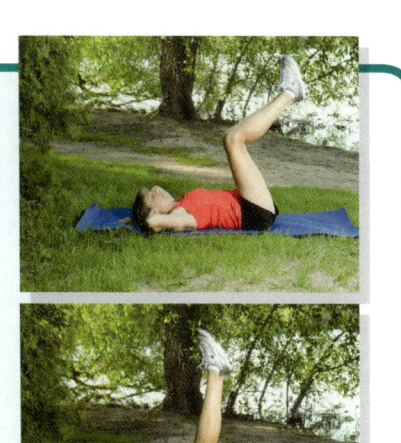

Four Weeks to Fabulous

Four Week Exercise Descriptions

Glider Back Lunge

Start on carpet and place glider under your right foot. Balance your weight mostly on your left foot, sliding your right foot and glider back behind you, bending your left knee and lunging. Return to starting position. Be careful not to overextend by lunging too far back.

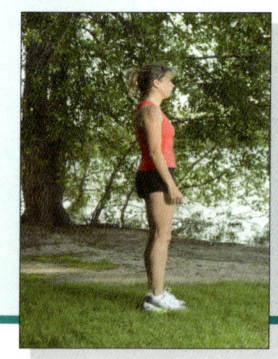

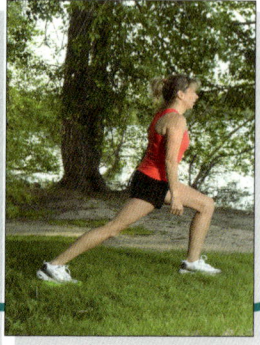

Band Straight-arm Pull Downs

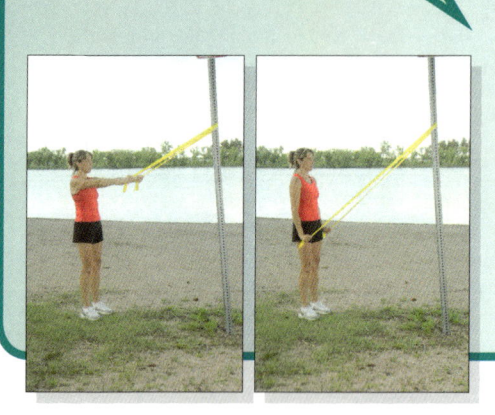

Wrap band around a post or object at or above eye level. Holding a handle or band end with each hand, face the object and then step back until you feel some resistance in the band. Arms should be extended out in front of you. Keeping palms down and arms straight, pull the band straight down to your sides, pause at full contraction, then return slowly to start.

Chapter 3: Four Weeks to Fabulous Physical Activity Plan

Band Standing Rows

Hold a handle in each hand and step onto the band with both feet. Leading the movement with your elbows, lift your elbows up to shoulder height, contracting your shoulder muscles. Return to starting position.

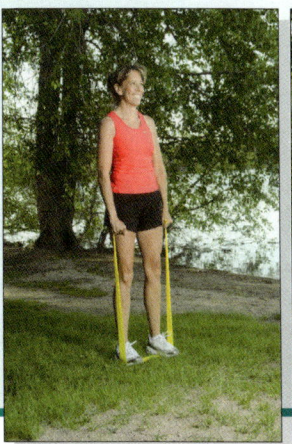

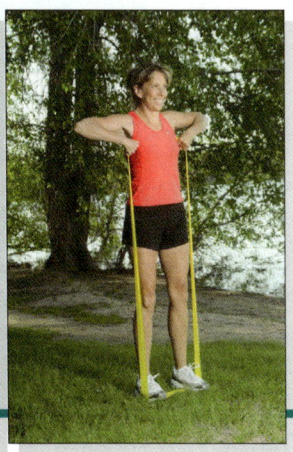

Four Weeks to Fabulous

Four Week Exercise Descriptions

Toe Stands

Stand twelve inches away from the back of a chair, with feet about twelve inches apart. Rest fingertips lightly on chair to help maintain balance as needed. Slowly raise yourself as high as possible on the balls of both feet. Remain on your toes for a count of three, breathing normally. Slowly lower yourself to starting position.

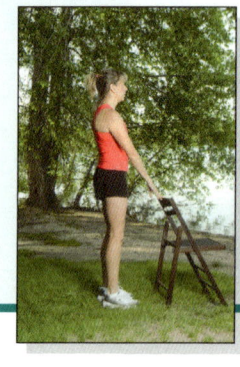

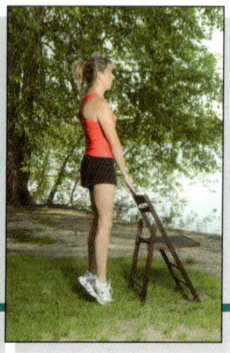

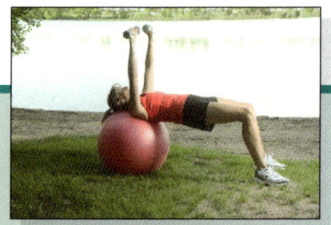

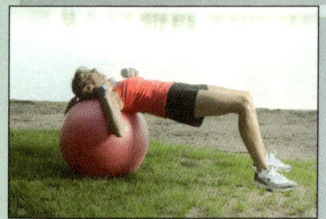

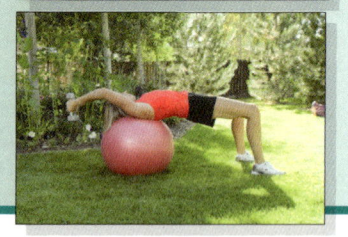

Ball Dumbbell Chest Press
(Progressing to Chest Press with Pullovers)

Lie supine on the ball with head and shoulders supported by the ball. Lift hips so your body forms a tabletop. Holding a dumbbell in each hand, extend your arms up toward the ceiling with the weights in line with your chest. Lower the weights to your chest, allowing your elbows to go out to the side; then extend your arms back up to the start. In later weeks, as you progress, add the pullovers. With arms extended up toward the ceiling, palms facing each other, elbows slightly bent, lower weight back over your head, the movement coming from your shoulders, NOT your elbows. Once you have reached a good stretch, slowly return to start.

Chapter 3: Four Weeks to Fabulous Physical Activity Plan

Axe Chop with Squats

Start with feet about hip-width apart, toes pointed straight ahead. Standing tall with dumbbell weight extended overhead in both hands, lower your body down to a squat, at the same time swinging the weight down between your legs simulating an ax chop. Keep your back straight and your eyes forward. As you return to the starting position, swing the weight back up overhead. Lean to one side with arms overhead, keeping back straight. Return weight to middle and repeat sequence, alternating sides when performing side-bends.

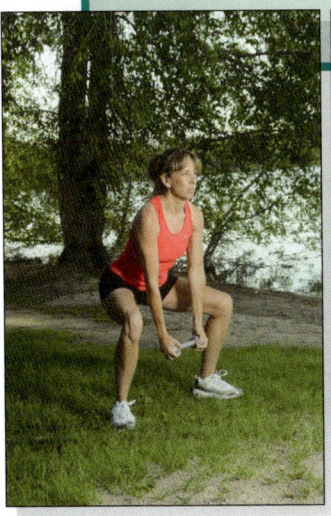

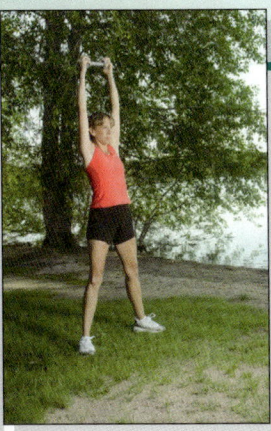

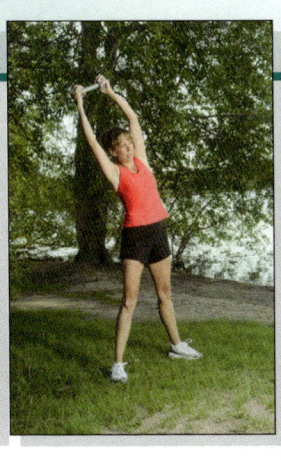

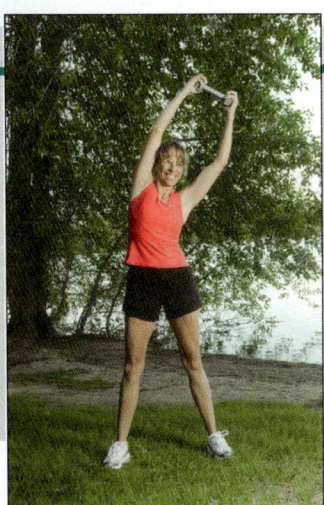

Four Weeks to Fabulous

Four Week Exercise Descriptions

Wide-stance Squat with Dumbbell

Stand with legs more than hip-width apart, toes turned out. Hold one dumbbell in both hands with the dumbbell in front of you. Keeping your back straight, squat without bending forward. Pause at the bottom of your squat then return to starting position.

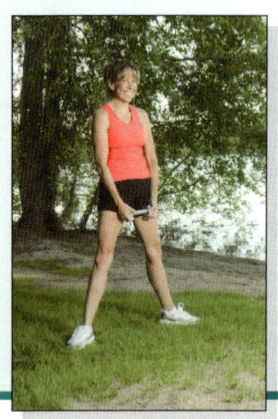

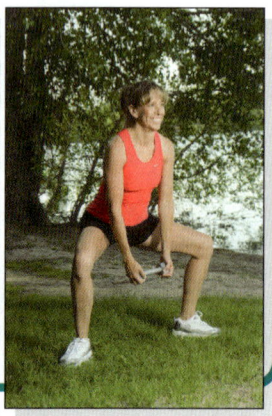

Ball Crunch

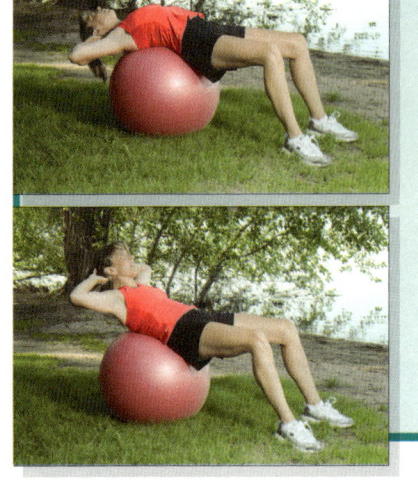

Sit upright on an exercise ball and walk your feet forward, letting the ball roll up on your spine until it is supporting your lower back. Your head and shoulders are off the ball, knees are in line with ankles, and feet are firmly on the floor. Place hands behind head and open elbows. Exhale and lift your head and shoulders forward so your rib cage moves closer to your hips, then pause. Inhale as you lower your head and shoulders back to starting position.

Chapter 3: Four Weeks to Fabulous Physical Activity Plan

Single-leg Chair Squats

Stand on one foot placing the other foot on a chair behind you. Stand tall, slowly squatting until your thigh is close to or parallel to the floor (being sure the knee of the working leg does not move forward beyond the toe). Push through the heel of the support leg and return to upright position.

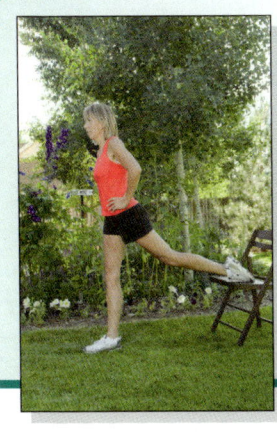

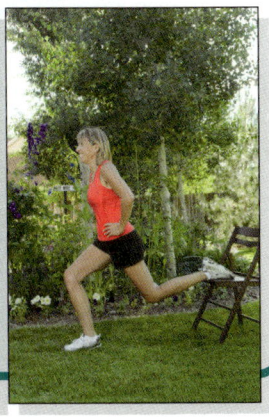

Side Crunch

Lie on your left side, legs out straight. Place your right hand behind your head and your left hand on your right obliques, or side muscles. Slowly contract your obliques while lifting your left shoulder two or six inches off the ground, being careful not to pull on your head and neck. Hold for one count and lower.

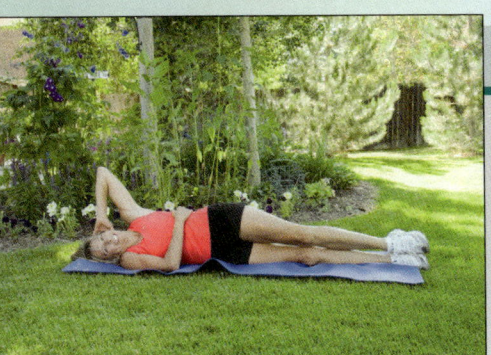

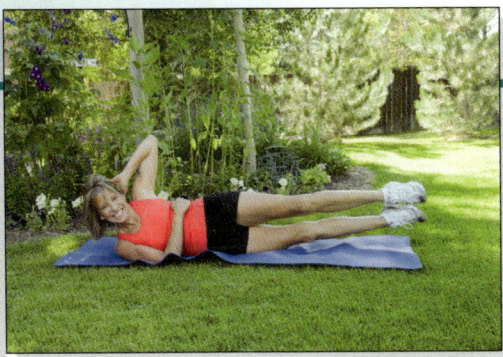

Glider Side Lunge

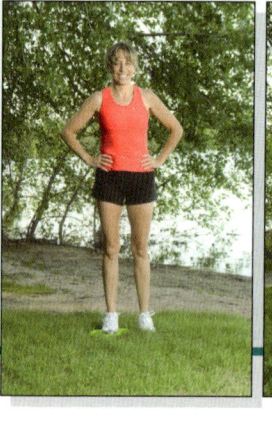

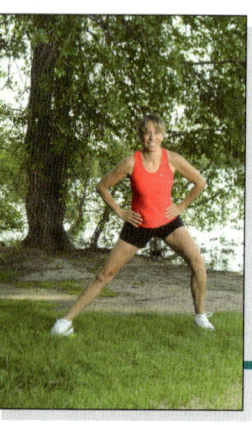

Start on carpet and place glider under your right foot. Balance your weight mostly on your left foot, sliding your right foot and glider out directly to the side and bending your left knee and lunging to the side. Return to starting position. Be careful not to overextend by lunging too far to the side.

Chapter 3: Four Weeks to Fabulous Physical Activity Plan

Week 1 Four Weeks to Fabulous
Beginner

	Endurance	Strength Training— No rest between exercises	Time or Repetitions
Monday & Friday "A man is not old until regrets take place of dreams." —John Barrymore	10-15 minutes fast-paced walking (may be used as warm-up)	Warm-up Chair Squats Band Rows (Palms Down to Palms Up) Dumbbell Hammer Curl to Shoulder Press Side Plank on Elbow Glider Back Lunge Band Straight-arm Pull Downs Band Standing Rows Ball Dumbbell Chest Press Ball Crunch Toe Stands	5 minutes 15 reps 15 reps 15 reps 15 seconds/side 10 reps/leg 10 reps 10 reps 10 reps 15 reps 30 seconds
Tuesday & Thursday "Build your weaknesses until they become your strengths." —Knute Rockne	20-30 minutes fast-paced walking		
Wednesday "We would accomplish many more things if we did not think of them as impossible." —Chretien Malesherbes	10-15 minutes fast-paced walking (may be used as warm-up)	Warm-up Wide-stance Squats with Dumbbells Band Rows (Palms Down) Ball Dumbbell Chest Press Band Bicep Curls Side Plank on Elbow Glider Back Lunge Band Standing Rows Band Straight-arm Pull Downs Ball Crunch Toe Stands	5 minutes 15 reps 15 reps 10 reps 15 reps 15 second/side 10 per leg 10 reps 10 reps 15 reps 30 seconds
Saturday "Opportunities are never lost; they are taken by others." —Source Unknown	20-30 minutes fast-paced walking		
Sunday "The future has a way of arriving unannounced." —George Will	Off or light activity		

Four Weeks to Fabulous

Week 2 *Four Weeks to Fabulous*
Beginner

	Endurance	Strength Training—No rest between exercises	Time or Repetitions
Monday & Friday "Our life is frittered away by detail. Simplify, simplify." —Henry David Thoreau	15-20 minutes fast-paced walking (may be used as warm-up)	Warm-up Wide-stance Squats with Dumbbells Band Rows (Palms Down) Ball Dumbbell Chest Press Band Bicep Curls Side Plank on Elbow Glider Back Lunge Band Standing Rows Band Straight-arm Pull Downs Ball Crunch Toe Stands ***Repeat circuit twice***	5 minutes 15 reps 15 reps 10 reps 15 reps 15 seconds/side 10 reps/leg 10 reps 10 reps 15 reps 30 seconds Increase resistance if appropriate.
Tuesday & Thursday "It's important to look at yourself and identify your gremlins." —Gary Mack	25-35 minutes fast-paced walking		
Wednesday "My philosophy is that not only are you responsible for your life, but doing the best at this moment puts you in the best place for the next moment." —Oprah Winfrey	15-20 minutes fast-paced walking (may be used as warm-up)	Warm-up Chair Squats Band Rows (Palms Down) Dumbbell Hammer Curl to Shoulder Press Side Plank on Elbow Glider Back Lunge Band Straight-arm Pull Downs Band Standing Rows Ball Dumbbell Chest Press Ball Crunch Toe Stands ***Repeat circuit twice***	5 minutes 15 reps 15 reps 15 reps 15 seconds/side 10 reps/leg 10 reps 10 reps 10 reps 15 reps 45 seconds Increase resistance if appropriate.
Saturday "It is our choices…that show what we truly are, far more than our abilities." —J. K. Rowling	25-35 minutes fast-paced walking		
Sunday "We've got two lives. The one we're given and the one that we make." —Kobe Yamada	Off or light activity		

Chapter 3: Four Weeks to Fabulous Physical Activity Plan

Week 3 Four Weeks to Fabulous
Beginner

	Endurance	Strength Training— No rest between exercises	Time or Repetitions
Monday & Friday "Health is beauty, and the most perfect health is the most perfect beauty." —William Shenstone	20-25 minutes fast-paced walking (may be used as warm-up)	Warm-up Chair Squats Band Rows (Palms Down to Palms Up) Dumbbell Hammer Curl to Shoulder Press Side Plank on Elbow Glider Back Lunge Band Straight-arm Pull Downs Band Standing Rows Ball Dumbbell Chest Press Ball Crunch Toe Stands ***Repeat circuit twice***	5 minutes 15 reps 15 reps each 15 reps 30 seconds/side 15 reps 15 reps 15 reps 15 reps 15 reps 1 minute Increase resistance if appropriate.
Tuesday & Thursday "Life is like a bicycle. To keep your balance you must keep moving." —Albert Einstein	35-45 minutes fast-paced walking Include Interval Workout.		
Wednesday "The race goes not always to the swift, but to those who keep on running." —Unknown	20-25 minutes fast-paced walking (may be used as warm-up)	Warm-up Wide-stance Squats with Dumbbells Band Rows (Palms Down) Ball Dumbbell Chest Press Band Bicep Curls Side Plank on Elbow Glider Back Lunge Band Standing Rows Band Straight-arm Pull Downs Ball Crunch Toe Stands ***Repeat circuit twice***	5 minutes 15 reps 15 reps 10 reps 15 reps 30 seconds/side 10 reps/leg 10 reps 10 reps 15 reps 30 seconds Increase resistance if appropriate.
Saturday "We cannot direct the wind, but we can adjust the sails." —Bertha Calloway	35-45 minutes fast-paced walking Include Interval Workout.		
Sunday "Never look where you're going. Always look where you want to go." —Bob Ernst	Off or light activity		

Four Weeks to Fabulous

Week 4 Four Weeks to Fabulous
Beginner

	Endurance	Strength Training—No rest between exercises	Time or Repetitions
Monday & Friday "The less tension and effort, the faster and more powerful you will be." —Bruce Lee	20-25 minutes fast-paced walking (may be used as warm-up)	Warm-up Wide-stance Squats with Dumbbells Band Rows (Palms Down to Palms Up) Ball Dumbbell Chest Press Band Bicep Curls Side Plank on Elbow to Down Plank Glider Back Lunge Band Standing Rows Band Straight-arm Pull Downs Ball Crunch Toe Stands ***Repeat circuit three times***	5 minutes 15 reps 15 reps 10 reps 15 reps 30 seconds/side 15 reps/leg 15 reps 15 reps 15 reps 1 minute Increase resistance if appropriate.
Tuesday & Thursday "Who looks outside, dreams. Who looks inside, awakens." —Carl Jung	45-55 minutes fast-paced walking		
Wednesday "Slumps are like a soft bed, easy to get into and hard to get out of." —Johnny Bench	20-25 minutes fast-paced walking (may be used as warm-up)	Warm-up Chair Squats Band Rows (Palms Down to Palms Up) Dumbbell Hammer Curl to Shoulder Press Side Plank on Elbow to Down Plank Glider Back Lunges Band Straight-arm Pull Downs Band Standing Rows Ball Dumbbell Chest Press Ball Crunch Toe Stands ***Repeat circuit three times***	5 minutes 15 reps 15 reps 15 reps 30 seconds/side 15 reps/leg 15 reps 15 reps 15 reps 15 reps 1 minute Increase resistance if appropriate.
Saturday "Victory is won not in miles but in inches. Win a little now, hold your ground, and later, win a little more." —Louis L'Amour	45-55 minutes fast-paced walking		
Sunday "Ninety percent of the game is half mental." —Yogi Berra	Off or light activity		

Chapter 3: Four Weeks to Fabulous Physical Activity Plan

Week 1 Four Weeks to Fabulous
Intermediate

	Endurance	Strength Training—No rest between exercises	Time or Repetitions
Monday & Friday "If you don't like something change it; if you can't change it, change the way you think about it." —Mary Engelbreit	15-20 minutes fast-paced walking (may be used as warm-up)	Warm-up Axe Chops with Squats Band Rows (Palms Down to Palms Up) Ball Dumbbell Chest Press Side Plank on Elbow Glider Back Lunge Toe Stands Band Straight-arm Pull Downs Band Standing Rows Dumbbell Hammer Curls to Shoulder Press Ball Crunch	5 minutes 15 reps 15 reps each 15 reps 30 seconds/side 10 reps/leg 45 seconds 15 reps 15 reps 15 reps 1 minute
Tuesday & Thursday "Jumping for joy is good exercise." —Unknown	25-30 minutes fast-paced walking Include Interval Workout.		
Wednesday "The principle is competing against yourself. It's about self-improvement, about being better than you were the day before." —Steve Young	15-20 minutes fast-paced walking (may be used as warm-up)	Warm-up Single-leg Chair Squat Band Straight-arm Pull Downs Ball Dumbbell Chest Press Side Crunch Glider Side Lunge Toe Stands Band Rows (Palms Down to Palms Up) Band Standing Rows Dumbbell Bicep Curls to Shoulder Press Reverse Crunch	5 minutes 10 reps 15 reps 15 reps 15 reps/side 10 reps/leg 45 seconds 15 reps each 15 reps 15 reps 1 minute
Saturday "Don't let yesterday's thoughts eat away at today's opportunities." —Unknown	25-35 minutes fast-paced walking Include Interval Workout.		
Sunday "We are what we repeatedly do. Excellence, then, is not an act, but a habit." —Aristotle	Off or light activity		

Four Weeks to Fabulous

Week 2 Four Weeks to Fabulous
Intermediate

	Endurance	Strength Training—No rest between exercises	Time or Repetitions
Monday & Friday "Be not afraid of going slowly; be afraid only of standing still." —Chinese Proverb	20-25 minutes fast-paced walking (may be used as warm-up)	Warm-up Single-leg Chair Squat Band Straight-arm Pull Downs Ball Dumbbell Chest Press Side Crunch Glider Side Lunge Toe Stands Band Rows (Palms Down to Palms Up) Band Standing Rows Dumbbell Bicep Curls to Shoulder Press Reverse Crunch	5 minutes 12 reps 15 reps 15 reps 15 reps/side 12 reps 1 minute 15 reps each 15 reps 15 reps 1 minute Increase resistance if appropriate.
Tuesday & Thursday "A man who wants something will find a way; a man who doesn't will find an excuse." —Stephan Dolley Jr.	35-40 minutes fast-paced walking Include Interval Workout.		
Wednesday "It actually takes more energy to deny dreams and desires than it does to pursue them." —Candy Paull	20-25 minutes fast-paced walking (may be used as warm-up)	Warm-up Axe Chops with Squats Band Rows (Palms Down to Palms Up) Ball Dumbbell Chest Press Side Plank on Elbows Glider Back Lunge Toe Stands Band Straight-arm Pull Downs Band Standing Rows Dumbbell Hammer Curls to Shoulder Press Ball Crunch	5 minutes 15 reps 15 reps each 15 reps 30 seconds/side 12 reps/leg 45 seconds 15 reps 15 reps 15 reps 1 minute Increase resistance if appropriate.
Saturday "Our actions are the spring of our happiness or misery." —Phillip Skelton	40-45 minutes fast-paced walking Include Interval Workout.		
Sunday "It is never too late to be what you might have been." —George Elliot	Off or light activity		

Chapter 3: Four Weeks to Fabulous Physical Activity Plan

Week 3 Four Weeks to Fabulous
Intermediate

	Endurance	Strength Training—No rest between exercises	Time or Repetitions
Monday & Friday "My business is not to remake myself, but to make the absolute best of what God made." —Robert Browning	25-30 minutes fast-paced walking (may be used as warm-up)	Warm-up Axe Chops w/Squats–Weight w/Overhead Side Bends Band Rows (Palms Down–Up–In) Ball Dumbbell Chest Press to Pullovers Side Plank on Elbow to Down Plank Glider Back Lunge Toe Stands Band Straight-arm Pull Downs Band Standing Rows Dumbbell Hammer Curls to Shoulder Press Ball Crunch ***Repeat circuit twice***	5 minutes 15 reps 15 reps each 15 reps each 30 sec/direction 15 reps/leg 1 minute 20 reps 20 reps 15 reps 1 minute Increase resistance if appropriate.
Tuesday & Thursday "It takes courage to grow up and turn out to be who you really are." —E.E. Cummings	40-45 minutes fast-paced walking Include Interval Workout.		
Wednesday "It is not the outer circumstances that dictate what you can become, but what you can become that will create circumstances you desire." —Candy Paull	25-30 minutes fast-paced walking (may be used as warm-up)	Warm-up Single-leg Chair Squat Band Straight-arm Pull Downs Ball Dumbbell Chest Press Side Crunch Glider Side Lunge Toe Stands Band Rows (Palms Down–Up–In) Band Standing Rows Dumbbell Hammer Curls to Shoulder Press Reverse Crunch ***Repeat circuit twice***	5 minutes 15 reps 20 reps 15 reps 15 reps per side 15 reps 1 minute 15 reps each 20 reps 15 reps 1 minute Increase resistance if appropriate.
Saturday "Sometimes you have to get worse before you get better." —Tom Watson	40-45 minutes fast-paced walking Include Interval Workout.		
Sunday "Nothing happens till something moves." —Albert Einstein	Off or light activity		

Four Weeks to Fabulous

Week 4 Four Weeks to Fabulous
Intermediate

	Endurance	Strength Training—No rest between exercises	Time or Repetitions
Monday & Friday "When the game is over I just want to look at myself in the mirror, win or lose, and know I gave it everything I had." —Joe Montana	30-35 minutes fast-paced walking (may be used as warm-up)	Warm-up Single-leg Chair Squat Band Straight-arm Pull Downs Ball Dumbbell Chest Press Side Crunch Glider Side Lunge Toe Stands Band Rows (Palms Down–Up–In) Band Standing Rows Dumbbell Hammer Curls to Shoulder Press Reverse Crunch ***Repeat circuit three times***	5 minutes 15 reps 20 reps 15 reps 20 reps/side 15 reps 1 minute 15 reps each 20 reps 15 reps 1 minute Increase resistance if appropriate.
Tuesday & Thursday "I may win and I may lose, but I will never be defeated." —Emmitt Smith	45-55 minutes fast-paced walking Include Interval Workout		
Wednesday "Don't worry about mistakes. Making things out of mistakes, that's creativity." —Peter Max	30-35 minutes fast-paced walking (may be used as warm-up)	Warm-up Axe Chops w/Squats–Weight w/Overhead Side Bends Band Rows (Palms Down–Up–In) Ball Dumbbell Chest Press to Pullovers Side Plank on Elbows to Down Plank Glider Back Lunge Toe Stands Band Straight-arm Pull Downs Band Standing Rows Dumbbell Hammer Curls to Shoulder Press Ball Crunch ***Repeat circuit three times***	5 minutes 15 reps 15 reps each 15 reps each 45 sec/direction 15 reps/leg 1 minute 20 reps 20 reps 15 reps 1 minute Increase resistance if appropriate.
Saturday "Have the courage to live your vision in spite of your fears." —Ken Carey	55-60 minutes fast-paced walking Include Interval Workout.		
Sunday "The kingdom of God is within you." —LUKE 17:21 (NIV)	Off or light activity		

Supercharge Your Workout with Interval Training

Interval training is an exercise technique used by elite athletes to boost speed, power and endurance. Establishing strong base-level fitness is a good idea before adding interval training to your endurance workout. If your body is ready for more challenge, add this routine to boost heart and lung strength and weight loss results.

Interval training keeps your heart rate at a higher level than exercising at a steady pace—and pushes your body to get stronger. Your body will not be anticipating the intensity, so it will burn more calories not only during the higher intensity bout—but also during the rest periods in between.

You can do interval training on a bike, any cardio machine, walking, running, or even in a pool. Try this program two to three times a week to shake up your routine, lose weight, add speed and power to your sport, or just to beat boredom. Don't forget to warm up well prior to beginning, and stretch after the workout.

Four Weeks to Fabulous

20-Minute Interval Program

Minutes	Intensity*
1:00-4:00	3-5
4:00-4:30	6
4:30-6:00	4
6:00-6:30	7
6:30-8:00	4
8:00-8:30	8
8:30-10:00	5
10:00-10:30	9
10:30-12:00	5
12:00-12:30	8
12:30-14:00	5
14:00-14:30	7
14:30-16:00	4
16:00-16:30	6
16:30-20:00	3-4

*Rate your intensity on a scale of 1 to 10.
1 is very, very light.
2-3 is light.
5-6 is somewhat hard but still enables you to talk fairly comfortably.
7-8 is hard.
9 is very, very hard.
10 is total exhaustion.

Resources

American College of Sports Medicine
www.acsm.org

American Council on Exercise
www.acefitness.org

American Dietetic Association
www.eatright.org

American Heart Association
www.americanheart.org

Center for Disease Control and Prevention
www.fruitsandveggiesmatter.gov

National Strength and Conditioning Association
www.nsca-lift.org

United States Department of Agriculture
www.usda.gov
www.nutrition.gov

These and other fun online health quizzes and wellness resources can be found at www.2BFIT.net.

About the Author

Alice Burron has been interviewed by national publications as a leading fitness expert, is the leading fitness expert for NurseTogether.com, and is an ACE personal trainer and corporate wellness expert. She earned a master's in physical education with an emphasis in exercise physiology from the University of Wyoming and is a leading local and national fitness expert. *Four Weeks to Fabulous* is her first book. Visit her on the web at www.2BFIT.net.

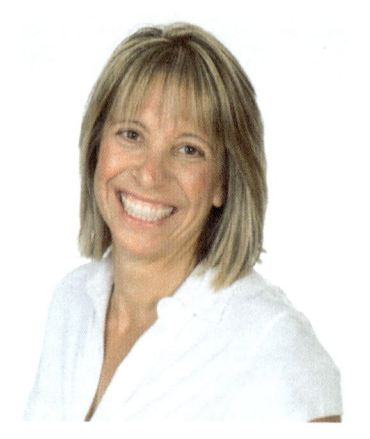

Additional books and bulk order discounts can be requested at info@2BFIT.net.

Acknowledgments

Four Weeks to Fabulous would still be just an idea in my head if it weren't for so many encouraging and gifted people to support me along the way.

My husband and four children have forever encouraged me to pursue my passion for my career in the wellness field, and to that I am so thankful. I am also so grateful to my wonderful parents who have always believed in me.

Mary Bushkuhl, personal trainer and massage therapist at Mary's Fitness, Cheyenne, Wyoming, was instrumental in designing the workout program. Thanks to Mary I never felt I was alone in this enormous project.

Sarah Morales, dietitian and soul-sister, came through for me like an angel for the nutritional analysis of the Four Weeks menus.

To my colleagues at Cheyenne Regional Medical Center, in Cheyenne, Wyoming, and the staff at Nursetogether.com; it has been a pleasure and honor to work with such dedicated professionals who truly care about the clients they serve.

Finally, thank you to those who tested the program and gave me valuable feedback. You helped me learn what was needed to make this book a success for every individual who embarks on the Four Weeks Journey.

Thank you all!

"The Lord will continually guide you; He will satisfy your needs...and will strengthen your frame. You will be like a well-watered garden, like a spring whose waters never fail." Isaiah 58:11

Made in the USA
Lexington, KY
23 February 2011